Third Space Endoscopy

Michael Ujiki • Zachary M. Callahan
Editors

Third Space Endoscopy

Springer

Editors
Michael Ujiki
General Surgery
NorthShore University Health System
Evanston, IL, USA

Zachary M. Callahan
Minimally Invasive Surgeon
and Surgical Endoscopist
The University of Tennessee Health
Science Center - Nashville Campus
Nashville, TN, USA

ISBN 978-3-031-84508-6 ISBN 978-3-031-84509-3 (eBook)
https://doi.org/10.1007/978-3-031-84509-3

This Springer imprint is published by the registered company Springer Nature Switzerland AG
The registered company address is: Gewerbestrasse 11, 6330 Cham, Switzerland

Preface

In 2008, Dr. Haruhiro Inoue performed the first PerOral Endoscopic Myotomy (POEM) on a human patient. This leap from animal models catapulted the field of advanced endoscopy into a novel, vast, and completely unknown territory. Access to a location between the intra- and extraluminal space razed the anatomical limitations of contemporary surgical treatments. Since its widespread adoption, POEM has changed the treatment algorithm of not just achalasia but numerous disorders affecting the gastrointestinal tract. These methods and techniques disseminated beyond benign disease and have solidly established a major role in numerous malignant conditions as well.

The text is organized into sections, exploring advanced endoscopic procedures with an emphasis on Third Space Endoscopy. These sections include Tissue Resection, Intentional Scar Formation, and Muscle Division. The authors are widely known and respected leaders in their respective fields. The chapters maintain an emphasis on procedural details, assisted by detailed diagrams and operative pictures.

We intend this book for both beginners and experts in the field, looking to augment their understanding and expertise of Third Space Endoscopy.

Third Space Endoscopy would not be possible without the editorial staff at Springer Nature including Responsible Editor Kristopher Spring. We are particularly grateful to Production Editor Sharath Rangaraj for his respectful persistence and attention to detail.

Evanston, IL, USA — Michael Ujiki
Nashville, TN, USA — Zachary M. Callahan

Contents

Contributors

Derrius Anderson University of Chicago Medicine, Chicago, IL, USA

Jamie Benson Department of Surgery, University Hospitals Cleveland Medical Center, Cleveland, OH, USA

Jerry T. Dang Department of General Surgery, Digestive Disease Institute, Cleveland Clinic, Cleveland, OH, USA

Kamil Erozkan Department of Colorectal Surgery, Digestive Disease and Surgery Institute, Cleveland Clinic, Cleveland, OH, USA

Lucas Fair Department of Minimally Invasive Surgery, Baylor University Medical Center, Dallas, TX, USA
Center for Advanced Surgery, Baylor Scott and White Health, Dallas, TX, USA
Research Institute, Dallas, TX, USA

Melissa M. Felinski Division of Minimally Invasive and Elective General Surgery, Department of Surgery, McGovern Medical School, University of Texas Health Science Center at Houston, Houston, TX, USA

Emre Gorgun Department of Colorectal Surgery, Digestive Disease and Surgery Institute, Cleveland Clinic, Cleveland, OH, USA

Mason Hedberg Department of Surgery, Endeavor Health, Evanston, IL, USA

Haruhiro Inoue Digestive Diseases Center, Showa University Koto Toyosu Hosptital, Tokyo, Japan

Andrew Kastenmeier Department of Surgery, Medical College of Wisconsin, Milwaukee, WI, USA

Monika A. Krezalek Department of Surgery, Division of Gastrointestinal and General Surgery, Section of Colon and Rectal Surgery, Endeavor Health, Evanston, IL, USA

Matthew Kroh Department of General Surgery, Digestive Disease Institute, Cleveland Clinic, Cleveland, OH, USA

Joshua Lyons Department of Surgery, University Hospitals Cleveland Medical Center, Cleveland, OH, USA

Jeffrey Marks Department of Surgery, University Hospitals Cleveland Medical Center, Cleveland, OH, USA

Oscar A. Olavarria Division of Minimally Invasive and Elective General Surgery, Department of Surgery, McGovern Medical School, University of Texas Health Science Center at Houston, Houston, TX, USA

Yaeji Park Department of General Surgery, The University of Chicago, Chicago, IL, USA

Kyle A. Perry Department of Surgery, Wexner Medical Center, The Ohio State University, Columbus, OH, USA

Shinil K. Shah Division of Minimally Invasive and Elective General Surgery, Department of Surgery, McGovern Medical School, University of Texas Health Science Center at Houston, Houston, TX, USA

Mayo Tanabe Digestive Diseases Center, Showa University Koto Toyosu Hospital, Tokyo, Japan

Peter A. Walker Division of Minimally Invasive and Elective General Surgery, Department of Surgery, McGovern Medical School, University of Texas Health Science Center at Houston, Houston, TX, USA

Marc A. Ward Department of Minimally Invasive Surgery, Baylor University Medical Center, Dallas, TX, USA
Center for Advanced Surgery, Baylor Scott and White Health, Dallas, TX, USA
Texas A&M College of Medicine, Bryan, TX, USA

Erik B. Wilson Division of Minimally Invasive and Elective General Surgery, Department of Surgery, McGovern Medical School, University of Texas Health Science Center at Houston, Houston, TX, USA

Joshua S. Winder Division of Minimally Invasive and Bariatric Surgery, Department of Surgery, Penn State Milton S. Hershey Medical Center, Hershey, PA, USA

Tarik K. Yuce Department of Surgery, Wexner Medical Center, The Ohio State University, Columbus, OH, USA

Chapter 1
History of Third Space Endoscopy

Joshua S. Winder

Introduction

Endoscopy has revolutionized surgery by offering minimally invasive techniques that improve patient outcomes and reduce recovery times. Among these advancements, third space endoscopy has emerged as a groundbreaking innovation, particularly in the field of submucosal endoscopic surgery (SES). This technique provides access to previously challenging anatomical areas, opening new possibilities for treating various gastrointestinal conditions. This chapter delves into the evolution of endoscopic surgery, the pivotal role of third space endoscopy, and its applications in SES.

A Brief History of Endoscopic Surgery

Early Beginnings

The concept of endoscopy dates back to the early nineteenth century when physicians first sought ways to explore the body's internal structures without the need for large incisions. In 1806, Philipp Bozzini, a German physician, developed the "Lichtleiter" (light conductor), a crude device used to examine the bladder [1, 2]. This rudimentary tool marked the dawn of endoscopic technology. The term "endoscope" is derived from the Greek words "endon" (inside) and "skopein" (to look),

J. S. Winder (✉)
Division of Minimally Invasive and Bariatric Surgery, Department of Surgery, Penn State Milton S. Hershey Medical Center, Hershey, PA, USA
e-mail: jwinder@pennstatehealth.psu.edu

M. Ujiki, Z. M. Callahan (eds.), *Third Space Endoscopy*,
https://doi.org/10.1007/978-3-031-84509-3_1

reflecting the core idea behind this approach. Despite its limitations, Bozzini's invention laid the groundwork for modern endoscopic tools [1].

Over the years, advances in light sources and optics gradually improved the practicality of endoscopy. By the early twentieth century, physicians were experimenting with flexible tubes and illumination techniques to peer into the human body [2]. Yet, significant challenges remained, particularly in terms of visualization and maneuverability.

Advancements in Technology

The twentieth century brought substantial progress in endoscopic technology. One of the most important breakthroughs came with the introduction of fiber optics in the 1950s, which drastically improved visualization inside the body [2, 3]. Fiber optics allowed light to be transmitted effectively into the body while enabling physicians to view internal structures more clearly. This revolutionized endoscopic procedures, giving rise to specialized scopes for different regions of the body, such as the gastrointestinal tract, bronchi, and abdomen. Instruments like the gastrointestinal endoscope, bronchoscope, and laparoscopy tools expanded the scope of endoscopic applications [3].

By the 1980s, endoscopic surgery began gaining traction as a minimally invasive alternative to traditional open surgery [2, 3]. Procedures like laparoscopic cholecystectomy, the removal of the gallbladder using small incisions and cameras, showcased the potential of these techniques. Minimally invasive surgery offered reduced recovery times, less postoperative pain, and shorter hospital stays, paving the way for widespread adoption across multiple surgical disciplines.

Emergence of Therapeutic Endoscopy

As endoscopy became more sophisticated, it transitioned from purely diagnostic purposes to therapeutic interventions [3]. Endoscopic techniques were developed for various gastrointestinal conditions, such as polypectomy, stenting, and the management of gastrointestinal bleeding. Endoscopic retrograde cholangiopancreatography (ERCP) and endoscopic mucosal resection (EMR) exemplify how endoscopy can be employed for both diagnosis and treatment.

Endoscopic techniques began to reduce the need for open surgeries, as patients benefited from less invasive methods. With innovations like stenting, dilation, and the management of gastrointestinal bleeding, endoscopy became a cornerstone of both diagnostic and therapeutic approaches, transforming the landscape of gastrointestinal surgery.

The Rise of Natural Orifice Transluminal Endoscopy Surgery (NOTES)

Emergence of Therapeutic Endoscopy

As endoscopy became more sophisticated, it transitioned from purely diagnostic purposes to therapeutic interventions. Endoscopic techniques were developed for various gastrointestinal conditions, such as polypectomy, stenting, and the management of gastrointestinal bleeding. ERCP and EMR exemplify how endoscopy can be employed for both diagnosis and treatment, reducing the need for invasive surgical interventions [4, 5]. Among these advancements, a significant experimental innovation that pushes the boundaries of minimally invasive techniques is natural orifice transluminal endoscopic surgery (NOTES).

NOTES and the Minimization of Surgical Trauma

The history of accessing the abdominal cavity for diagnostic and therapeutic purposes has evolved significantly over time. Traditional approaches, such as laparotomy, required large incisions to expose the area, but the introduction of minimally invasive laparoscopic techniques marked a major shift in reducing the morbidity associated with surgeries. Despite the advantages, laparoscopic surgery still carries risks like wound infections, hernias, and postsurgical pain due to skin incisions. To address these complications, *natural orifice transluminal endoscopic surgery (NOTES)* has emerged as a groundbreaking alternative, utilizing natural orifices like the mouth, anus, or vagina to access the abdominal cavity without external incisions [4, 5].

NOTES eliminates the need for external abdominal incisions, reducing complications such as surgical site infections (SSIs) and hernias that often arise from traditional surgical methods [4]. This technique reflects the culmination of centuries of endoscopic innovation, starting with Bozzini's invention of the rigid endoscope in 1805 and evolving through multiple technological advancements, including the fiber optic endoscope in the mid-twentieth century [2, 3, 5]. By enabling incisionless surgeries, NOTES provides distinct advantages in reducing adhesions and minimizing recovery time. Furthermore, it offers benefits for special populations, such as children and the morbidly obese, who may be more vulnerable to the complications of traditional surgery.

Challenges and Future Prospects of NOTES

Despite its potential, significant challenges hindered the widespread adoption of NOTES in human clinical practice. Technical difficulties, such as ensuring safe viscerotomy closure, improving the articulation of endoscopic devices, and managing contamination risks from nonsterile orifices, were a few of the many obstacles [5–7]. The development of specialized instruments and stronger collaboration between gastroenterology and surgical fields are critical to overcoming these challenges. Professional organizations, such as the Natural Orifice Surgery Consortium for Assessment and Research (NOSCAR), played a crucial role in advancing research and addressing both technical and societal aspects of this evolving field [5–7].

Although NOTES never took off as the paradigm-shifting surgical platform that many predicted, many of the principles and techniques that were developed and perfected as a result have translated into other areas of endoscopic surgery.

The Rise of Submucosal Endoscopic Surgery

Defining Submucosal Endoscopic Surgery

Submucosal endoscopic surgery (SES) refers to a subset of endoscopic procedures that target lesions located beneath the mucosal layer of the gastrointestinal tract. This approach enables the removal of submucosal tumors and lesions with minimal disruption to the surrounding tissue. SES techniques have gained prominence for their ability to provide effective treatment while minimizing complications and recovery time.

Historical Context and Development

The advent of SES can be traced back to the need for more effective methods of treating submucosal lesions, which were often challenging to access and remove using traditional endoscopic techniques [8, 9]. Early attempts at SES involved techniques such as needle knife dissection, which allowed for the resection of superficial lesions. However, these methods were limited by their potential for complications and suboptimal outcomes.

The introduction of endoscopic submucosal dissection (ESD) in the 1990s marked a significant milestone in SES [8]. Developed in Japan, ESD allowed for en bloc resection of larger lesions by dissecting the submucosal layer using specialized instruments. This technique offered greater precision and reduced recurrence rates compared to previous methods, thus garnering attention and adoption worldwide.

Transition to Third Space Endoscopy

Defining Third Space Endoscopy

Third space endoscopy refers to procedures that access the "third space," which is the anatomical area located between the mucosal and muscular layers of the gastrointestinal tract [8–10]. This innovative approach allows for greater access to submucosal structures, facilitating the treatment of a wide range of lesions and conditions.

The Conceptual Shift

The conceptual shift toward third space endoscopy emerged from the recognition of the limitations of traditional endoscopic techniques in accessing submucosal lesions. With the increasing complexity of gastrointestinal pathologies, there was a growing need for endoscopic approaches that could provide deeper access while minimizing surgical trauma.

The introduction of techniques such as peroral endoscopic myotomy (POEM) for treating achalasia highlighted the potential of third space endoscopy [9, 10]. By accessing the submucosal layer, surgeons could perform myotomy with minimal disruption to the surrounding tissue, resulting in shorter recovery times and fewer complications.

Key Innovations

Key innovations that facilitated the transition to third space endoscopy include:

1. Endoscopic ultrasound (EUS): The integration of EUS into endoscopic procedures allowed for precise localization of submucosal lesions, aiding in the planning and execution of third space surgeries.
2. Specialized instruments: The development of dedicated endoscopic instruments, such as the dual-channel endoscope and specialized dissection knives, provided the necessary tools for navigating and operating within the third space [5].
3. Training and techniques: The establishment of structured training programs and the sharing of techniques among practitioners contributed to the rapid adoption of third space endoscopy. Collaborative efforts through workshops and online resources helped standardize procedures and improve outcomes.

The Role of Third Space Endoscopy in Submucosal Endoscopic Surgery

Expanding Indications

Third space endoscopy has expanded the indications for SES beyond the removal of benign tumors. Conditions such as submucosal gastrointestinal stromal tumors (GISTs), achalasia, gastric outlet obstruction, and even certain cancers can now be addressed using third space techniques [8–10]. This has transformed the landscape of gastrointestinal surgery, offering patients less invasive options with reduced hospital stays.

Procedural Techniques

Several key procedural techniques have emerged within the realm of third space endoscopy:

- Peroral endoscopic myotomy (POEM): This technique allows for the treatment of achalasia by creating a myotomy in the submucosal space, alleviating dysphagia and improving patient quality of life. This technique has been adapted into treatment for other areas along the GI tract, most notably for gastric outlet obstruction with the use of peroral endoscopic pyloromyotomy (POP).
- Endoscopic submucosal dissection (ESD): ESD has been adapted to third space procedures, enabling the removal of larger submucosal lesions with increased precision and lower recurrence rates.
- Endoscopic mucosal resection (EMR): When combined with third space access, EMR can be used for complex lesions that require a more comprehensive approach.

Safety and Efficacy

The safety and efficacy of third space endoscopy have been supported by a growing body of literature. Studies have demonstrated that these techniques result in lower complication rates, shorter recovery times, and improved overall outcomes when compared to traditional surgical approaches [8–10].

Challenges and Future Directions

Technical Challenges

Despite its advantages, third space endoscopy is not without challenges. The complexity of these procedures requires a high level of skill and experience, and there is a learning curve associated with mastering the techniques. Additionally, complications such as perforation and bleeding can occur, necessitating the development of strategies to mitigate these risks.

Future Innovations

The future of third space endoscopy is promising, with ongoing research and innovation aimed at enhancing procedural safety and efficacy. Potential advancements include:

1. Robotic-assisted endoscopy: The integration of robotic systems could improve precision and control during complex procedures, allowing for more intricate dissection and resection [11].
2. Artificial intelligence (AI): AI algorithms could assist in lesion detection, characterization, and procedural planning, further enhancing the capabilities of third space endoscopy.
3. Training simulators: The development of advanced training simulators could provide practitioners with realistic practice scenarios, helping to bridge the gap between theoretical knowledge and practical skills.

Conclusion

The journey from traditional endoscopic surgery to third space endoscopy represents a significant evolution in the field of minimally invasive surgery. By enabling access to submucosal structures, third space techniques have transformed the treatment of gastrointestinal lesions, offering patients safer and more effective options. As technology continues to advance and techniques are refined, the future of third space endoscopy holds great promise for both patients and practitioners, paving the way for continued innovation in surgical care.

As we move forward, it is crucial to foster collaboration among healthcare professionals, researchers, and educators to ensure the continued growth and advancement of this transformative field. The history of endoscopic surgery is a testament to the power of innovation, and the emergence of third space endoscopy is a shining example of how far we have come and how far we can still go.

References

1. Doglietto F, Prevedello DM, Jane JA, Han J, Laws ER. Brief history of endoscopic transsphenoidal surgery – from Philipp Bozzini to the First World Congress of Endoscopic Skull Base Surgery. Neurosurg Focus. 2005;19(6) Available from: https://pubmed.ncbi.nlm.nih.gov/16398480/
2. Berci G, Forde KA. History of endoscopy: what lessons have we learned from the past? Surg Endosc. 2000;14(1):5–15.
3. Litynski GS. Endoscopic surgery: the history, the pioneers. World J Surg. 1999;23(8):745–53.
4. McGee MF, Rosen MJ, Marks J, Onders RP, Chak A, Faulx A, Chen VK, Ponsky J. A primer on natural orifice transluminal endoscopic surgery: building a new paradigm. Surg Innov. 2006;13(2):86–93.
5. Autorino R, Yakoubi R, White WM, Gettman M, De Sio M, Quattrone C, et al. Natural orifice transluminal endoscopic surgery (NOTES): where are we going? A bibliometric assessment. BJU Int. 2013;111(1):11–6.
6. Pauli EM, Ponsky JL. A modern history of the surgeon-endoscopist. Tech Gastrointest Endosc. 2013;15(4):166–72.
7. Pauli EM, Moyer MT, Haluck RS, Mathew A. Self-approximating transluminal access technique for natural orifice transluminal endoscopic surgery: a porcine survival study (with video). Gastrointest Endosc. 2008;67(4):690–7.
8. Fukuzawa M, Gotoda T. History of endoscopic submucosal dissection and role for colorectal endoscopic submucosal dissection: a Japanese perspective. Gastrointest Interv. 2012;1(1):30–5.
9. Pescarus R, Shlomovitz E, Swanstrom LL. Per-Oral endoscopic myotomy (POEM) for esophageal achalasia. Curr Gastroenterol Rep. 2014;16(1)
10. Nabi Z, Reddy DN. Third-space endoscopy: recent updates. J Dig Endosc. 2021;12(03):160–6.
11. Kim SH, Choi HS, Keum B, Chun HJ. Robotics in gastrointestinal endoscopy. Appl Sci (Switzerland). 2021;11(23)

Part I
Tissue Removal

Chapter 2
Endoscopic Mucosal Resection (EMR)

Yaeji Park and Monika A. Krezalek

Background [1–4]

- Endoscopic mucosal resection (EMR) was developed with the goal of minimally invasive and organ-sparing treatment of benign and early malignant gastrointestinal lesions. The technique was developed in Japan with the first indication for use in treatment of early gastric cancer. The use of EMR has since expanded to treat select superficial sessile lesions in the esophagus, duodenum, stomach, colon, and rectum.
- When compared to standard polypectomy, EMR allows for a wider and deeper specimen resection. It has the advantage of providing en bloc resection of lesions up to 2.5 cm in size. EMR also provides local staging for superficial gastrointestinal lesions, while local ablative therapies do not.
- EMR is more widely available than more advanced endoscopic procedures such as endoscopic submucosal dissection (ESD) or endoscopic full thickness resection (EFTR). EMR is associated with shorter procedural time and lesser morbidity when compared to ESD, EFTR, and surgical resection techniques. A disadvantage of EMR in treatment of larger lesions is that piecemeal resection may preclude the assessment of margins. Therefore, in cases of early malignant lesions, ESD may be the preferred method of treatment.

Y. Park
Department of General Surgery, The University of Chicago, Chicago, IL, USA
e-mail: Yaeji.Park@uchicagomedicine.org

M. A. Krezalek (✉)
Department of Surgery, Division of Gastrointestinal and General Surgery, Section of Colon and Rectal Surgery, Endeavor Health, Evanston, IL, USA
e-mail: mkrezalek@northshore.org

M. Ujiki, Z. M. Callahan (eds.), *Third Space Endoscopy*,
https://doi.org/10.1007/978-3-031-84509-3_2

Indications [2–5]

- Dysplastic superficial lesions without an invasive component are ideal for treatment with EMR. These include Barrett's esophagus–associated dysplasia, duodenal adenomas, large colorectal adenomas, and sessile serrated lesions.
- Select superficial lesions with limited submucosal invasion and absence of high-risk histologic features can also be treated with EMR. These, in general, have very low risk of lymph node involvement or distant spread and thus can potentially be managed endoscopically with curative intent, minimizing morbidity. High-risk histologic features include greater depth of submucosal invasion, lymphovascular invasion, perineural invasion, high tumor budding score, positive margins, or inability to assess margins due to piecemeal resection or cautery artifact.
- Early malignancies that can be treated with EMR in select patients include superficial esophageal cancer, superficial gastric cancer, superficial colorectal cancer, and small and low-risk gastric or colorectal neuroendocrine tumors. However, rates of en bloc resection are better and recurrence rates are lower with use of ESD when compared to EMR for treatment of malignant lesions.
- Larger lesions with suspected invasive component may be best served with upfront ESD as attempts at EMR cause submucosal scarring and may preclude future advanced endoscopic resection attempts.

Patient Evaluation [2–9]

Initial Evaluation

- It is important to assess the appropriateness and feasibility of EMR. Large lesions with high suspicion of malignancy or a biopsy-proven malignant component that invades submucosa should be recommended for ESD or surgical resection. Removal of lesions 20 mm or larger is considered technically difficult and in general requires advanced polyp resection technique and expertise. In general, en bloc removal is prefered and possible for lesions up to 25 mm when using EMR. Larger lesions will likely require piecemeal resection when decision is made to proceed with EMR.
- Location guides difficulty of resection. Duodenal lesions are most difficult to resect due to the thin wall and decreased scope mobility. Cecal lesions are also difficult to resect due to the thin wall; however, maneuverability of the endoscope is technically easier in the colon than in the duodenum and perforation is easier to manage comparatively.

Diagnostic Studies/Lesion Classification

- Endoscopic evaluation with assessment of lesion size can determine the likelihood of malignancy and difficulty of resection.
  - Polyp size and risk of malignancy:
    - <5 mm: Unlikely malignant
    - 6–15 mm: 2% risk
    - 16–25 mm: 19% risk
    - 26–35 mm: 43% risk
    - >35 mm: 76% risk
- Deep submucosa invasive cancer can be predicted by endoscopic evaluation using the Narrow-Band Imaging International Colorectal Endoscopic (NICE) classification, Japanese Narrow Band Imaging Expert Team (JNET) classification, Kudo classification, or Paris classification:
  - NICE and JNET classification use color variation and vascular pattern to predict submucosal invasion:
    - Type 1: Similar color or lighter than the background, uniform dark or white spots on the surface, most likely hyperplastic or sessile serrated polyps.
    - Type 2: Darker than background, brown vessels with oval, tubular, or branched white structures on the surface, most likely conventional adenoma or superficial submucosal invasion. JNET further divides into type 2A and type 2 B based on regular versus irregular vessel and surface pattern to distinguish low-grade versus high-grade dysplasia/invasive cancer.
    - Type 3: Dark lesions, disrupted or missing vessels forming an amorphous surface pattern or no pattern at all, most likely deep submucosal invasion.
- Kudo classification uses surface pit pattern to predict submucosal invasion:
  - Type I: Round pit, most likely benign normal mucosa.
  - Type II: Asteroid pit, most likely hyperplastic.
  - Type III-S: Small tubular or round pit, most likely tubular adenoma, dysplastic changes with 4% risk of invasion.
  - Type III-L: Large tubular or round pit, most likely tubular adenoma, dysplastic changes with 4% risk of invasion.
  - Type IV: Dendritic or gyrus-like pit, most likely tubulovillous or villous adenoma, dysplastic changes with 5% risk of invasion.
  - Type V-I: Nonstructured or amorphous pit, most likely invasive, dysplastic changes with 56% risk of invasion.
  - Type V-N: Decrease of amorphous pits or loss of pit, most likely invasive, dysplastic changes with 56% risk of invasion.

- The Paris classification uses morphologic features of the polyp such as depression and ulceration to estimate the risk of invasive cancer. The stages are listed in order of increasing risk of submucosal invasion:
  - Is: Sessile.
  - IIa: Slightly elevated.
  - IIb: Flat.
  - IIc: Slightly depressed.
  - III: Ulcerated.
- Other morphologic features used to assess the risk of invasive component include laterally spreading tumors with granular and nongranular surface appearance. Even-sized nodules in granular lesions have a < 2% risk of invasion. Mixed size nodules in granular lesions have up to 38% risk of invasion. Nongranular lesions have up to 40% risk of invasion.
- Despite all of the above classification methods, the interobserver agreement on the risk of invasion is modest at best. According to a multicenter video-based survey study, only 61% of endoscopists are able to accurately identify lesions with invasive adenocarcinoma as malignant. Nearly one in five rectal polyps diagnosed as adenoma clinically and on biopsy will harbor invasive adenocarcinoma.

Techniques

Planning

- EMR can be performed under sedation or monitored anesthesia care in the Gastroenterology suite if done as part of routine screening or therapeutic endoscopy. Conversely, EMR can also be performed under general anesthesia in the operating room for more complex lesions or as part of other surgical intervention.
- The patient is placed on the cart or OR table in standard position depending on the location of the lesion in the GI tract, secured, and with all pressure points padded.
- DVT prophylaxis in the form of SCDs +/− subcutaneous heparin is used if general anesthesia is used.
- Prophylactic antibiotics are generally not necessary.
- Numerous agents can be used for submucosal injection including normal saline (inexpensive, dissipates quickly), hypertonic saline (inexpensive, can cause tissue damage and inflammation), albumin (expensive, creates a longer lasting cushion), dextrose <15% in water (inexpensive, creates long-lasting cushion, can cause tissue damage and has increased risk of post-polypectomy syndrome), hyaluronic acid (expensive, creates a longer-lasting cushion, can promote tumor

cell growth), succinylated gelatin (inexpensive, creates a long lasting cushion), and synthetic commercial solutions with bulking agents, emulsifiers, and methylene blue (expensive, create a longer-lasting cushion, some may be proinflammatory).

- Dilute epinephrine (1:100,000) can be added to the injectate to reduce bleeding and increase the duration of the cushion.
- Methylene blue or indigo carmine can be added to the injectate to improve identification of the submucosal plane and margins.

Injection-Assisted EMR Steps (Fig. 2.1)

- Submucosal injection of a lifting solution creates a safety cushion. This method lifts the lesion away from the muscularis propria, minimizing risk of deeper injury and perforation.
- The lesion is removed with a snare (cold or hot) and can be resected as a single specimen or piecemeal for larger lesions.

Cap-Assisted EMR Steps (Fig. 2.2)

- Submucosal injection of a lifting solution creates a safety cushion.
- A cap is affixed to the end of the scope. A single-use mucosectomy device with a crescent-shaped electrocautery snare is positioned within the cap.
- The target lesion is suctioned into the cap and resected with the hot snare.
- Various shapes and sizes of caps exist. Caps can be soft or hard, straight, or oblique. Outer diameter of the cap ranges from 12.9 to 18 mm.

Ligation-Assisted EMR Steps (Fig. 2.3)

- Submucosal injection may be used, but is not necessary.
- A band ligation device is attached to the scope. The lesion is suctioned into the device, and the band is deployed creating a pseudopolyp.
- A hot snare is used to resect the lesion which can be done above or below the band.
- Each device is equipped with six bands for resection of multiple lesions.
- Ligating caps are available in two sizes to fit scopes of 9.5–13 mm and 11–14 mm diameter.

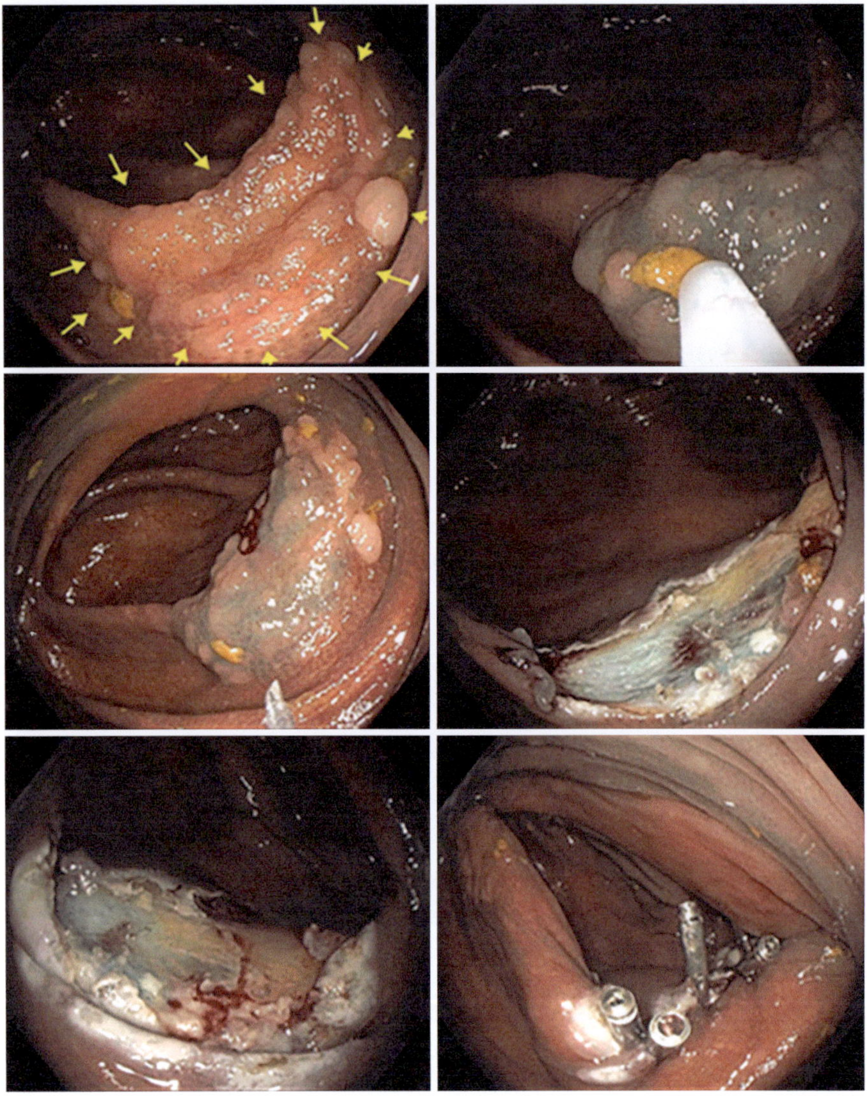

Fig. 2.1 Injection-assisted EMR of a 3 cm proximal ascending colon laterally spreading polyp. Resection was performed in a piecemeal fashion using snare cautery. The edges of the resection were ablated using the tip of the snare and cautery. Mucosal defect was closed using clips. (Images courtesy of Dr. Eric Elton)

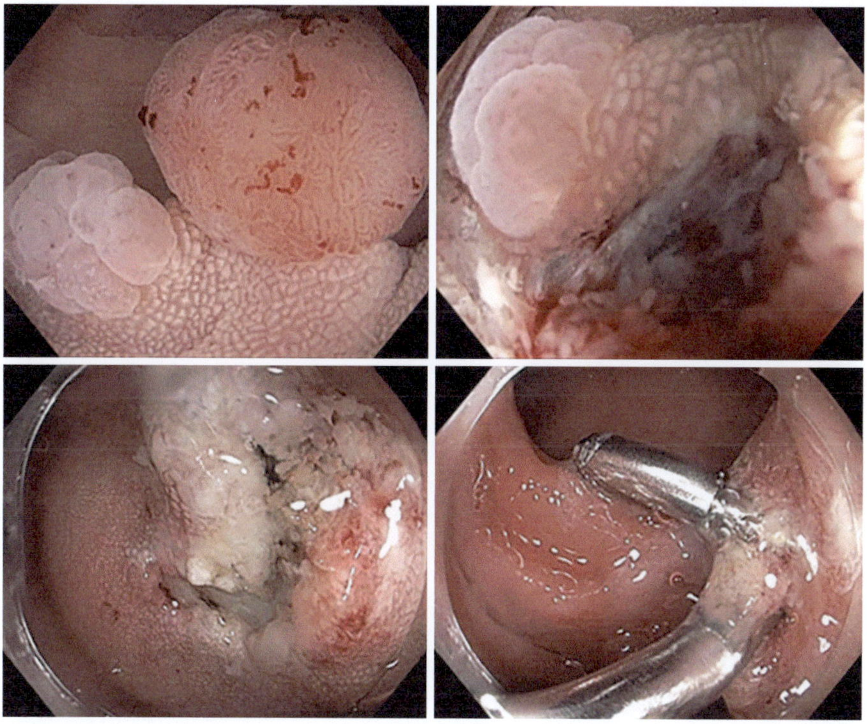

Fig. 2.2 Cap-assisted EMR of a 15 mm sigmoid colon polyp. Thermal marking with the tip of a snare was performed to mark the borders of the lesion. Polyp was suctioned into the cap and snare resection was performed. Base and edges of the defect were fulgurated using the tip of the snare. Defect was closed with hemostatic clips. (Images courtesy of Dr. Farhan Quader)

Underwater EMR Steps

- The bowel lumen is suctioned and collapsed, followed by instillation of water.
- This technique avoids overdistention of the wall of the bowel, effectively lifting the lesion off of the deeper bowel wall layers and can be helpful for non-lifting lesions due to scarring from prior procedure attempts (Fig. 2.4).
- No submucosal injection is required.
- This method has higher complete macroscopic resection rates, lower rates of recurrence, and no difference in immediate/delayed bleeding or perforation rate when compared to other EMR techniques.

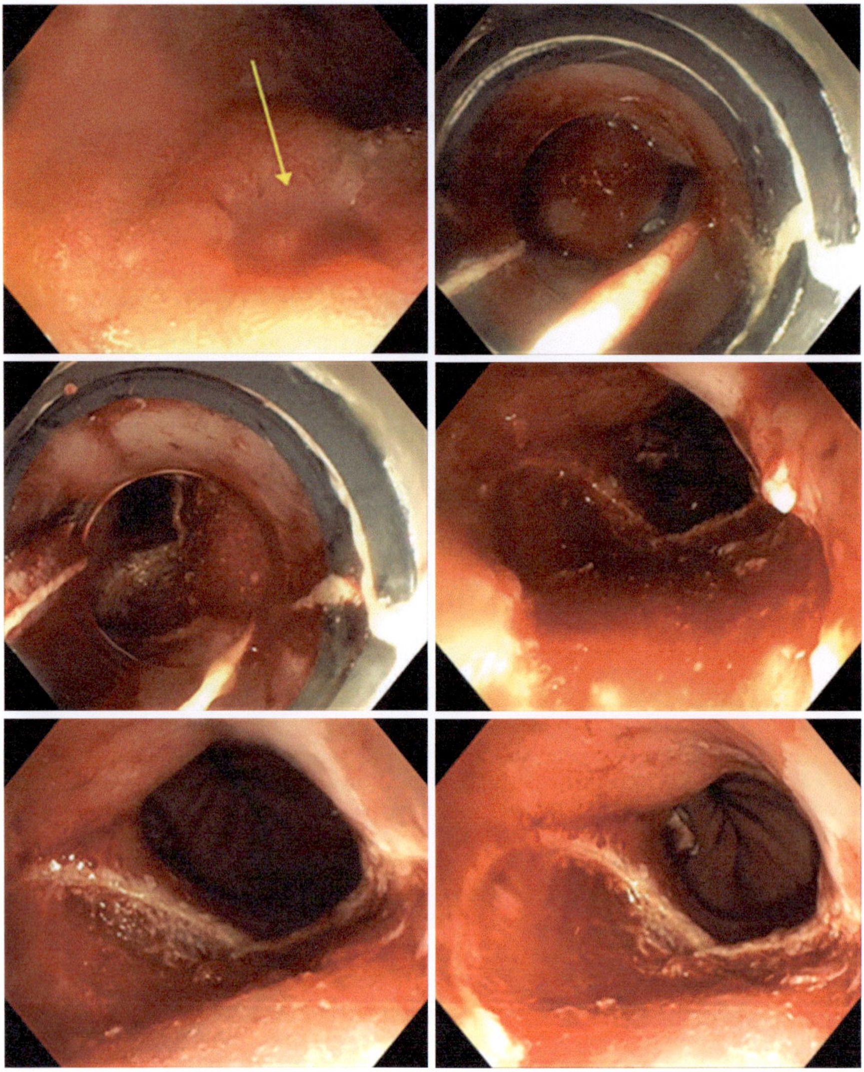

Fig. 2.3 Depressed lesion with adjacent ulceration in the background of Barrett's esophagus resected using ligation-assisted EMR. (Images courtesy of Dr. Eric Elton)

Postoperative Care/Surveillance

- Lesions 10 mm or larger removed en bloc with negative margins and no invasive component need repeat colonoscopy in 3 years.
- Polyps removed piecemeal, with positive margin, or inability to assess the margin need shorter follow-up interval in 3–6 months.

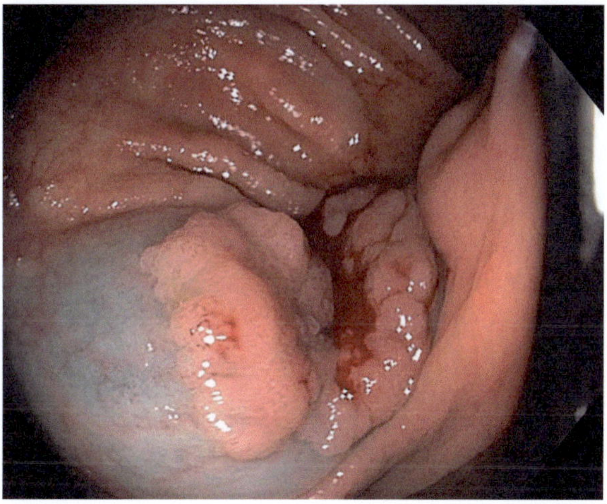

Fig. 2.4 Cecal sessile polyp after submucosal injection. Central portion of the lesion did not lift well due to scarring from prior attempt at removal

- Invasive cancer noted in a polyp requires standard staging studies, formal surgical consultation, and multidisciplinary tumor board discussion.

Outcomes [1–4, 10, 11]

EMR Based on Location and Indication

- Reported mean time to completion of EMR for large gastric lesions is 25.8+/−25.9 min, compared to 84.0+/−54.6 min for ESD.
- Barrett's esophagus-associated neoplasia:
  - No high-risk features: 98.8% complete eradication.
  - High-risk features present: 80.4% complete eradication.
  - Recurrence rate: 1.4%.
  - Bleeding rate: 1.2%.
  - Perforation rate: <0.5%.
  - Stenosis rate in circumferential EMR: 41–88%.
  - EMR + radiofrequency ablation:
    - Remission in 90% of patients at 5 years but 58% need additional thermal ablation.
- Superficial squamous cell cancer of the esophagus.
  - En bloc resection rate: 49.3% (vs. 97.1% with ESD).
  - Recurrence rate: 11.5% (vs. 0.3% with ESD).
- Early gastric cancer.

    - Recurrence rate: 6.4% (vs. 0.7% with ESD).
- Gastric carcinoid.
    - Slightly lower rate of complete resection compared to ESD.
    - Similar recurrence rate and survival rate.
- Non-ampullary duodenal adenomas:
    - 70–96% success rate
    - 83% complete resection with underwater EMR
    - However, high risk of delayed bleeding, water intoxication syndrome, stricture formation.
- Colon.
    - Recurrence rate: 3% (en bloc resection) vs. 20% (piecemeal resection).
    - Intraprocedural bleeding rate: 11–22% (>20 mm lesions).
    - Postprocedural bleeding rate: 2–11%.
    - Perforation rate: <1%.

Pitfall	Pearl
Positive margin or margin cannot be assessed	Delineate the margins of the lesion prior to any manipulation or injection as these can become obscured during the procedure. Margin of resection can be marked with cautery to ensure adequate margins (hot snare, APC probe) Specimen should be oriented and mounted (pinned) to a board prior to fixation to prevent folding of the edges and aid in pathologic examination of margins
Positive deep margin or depth of invasion cannot be assessed based on the amount of submucosa present	Avoid attempts at EMR for lesions that would be better removed by ESD Invasive lesions will show non-lifting sign during injection, typically reflective of the fact that the lesion cannot be removed endoscopically. EMR should not be attempted if non-lifting is thought to be related to deep invasion EMR can be attempted if non-lifting is suspected to be due to fibrosis from prior attempts at biopsy or removal (Fig. 2.4). Underwater technique is very useful in this situation
Perforation or bleeding	Specimen and resection bed should be examined (Fig. 2.5). Evidence of deep resection of the muscularis propria (target sign) should be identified early and the defect should be closed Clips and endoscopic suturing devices should be readily available

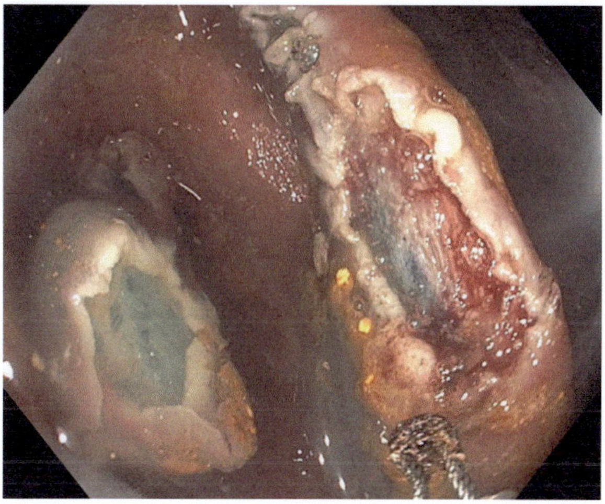

Fig. 2.5 Injection-assisted EMR of a cecal polyp. The specimen and resection bed are examined side by side showing a clean cut surface without any evidence of deeper resection. (Image courtesy of Dr. Eric Elton)

References

1. Soetikno RM, Gotoda T, Nakanishi Y, Soehendra N. Endoscopic mucosal resection. Gastrointest Endosc. 2003;57(4):567–79. Available from: https://pubmed.ncbi.nlm.nih.gov/12665775/
2. Mannath J, Ragunath K. Endoscopic mucosal resection: who and how? Ther Adv Gastroenterol. 2011;4(5):275. Available from: /pmc/articles/PMC3165204/
3. Hwang JH, Konda V, Abu Dayyeh BK, Chauhan SS, Enestvedt BK, Fujii-Lau LL, et al. Endoscopic mucosal resection. Gastrointest Endosc. 2015;82(2):215–26. Available from: https://pubmed.ncbi.nlm.nih.gov/26077453/
4. Shaukat A, Kaltenbach T, Dominitz JA, Robertson DJ, Anderson JC, Cruise M, et al. Endoscopic recognition and management strategies for malignant colorectal polyps: recommendations of the US multi-society task force on colorectal cancer. Am J Gastroenterol. 2020;115(11):1751–67. Available from: https://pubmed.ncbi.nlm.nih.gov/33156093/
5. Thiruvengadam SS, Fung BM, Barakat MT, Tabibian JH. Endoscopic mucosal resection: best practices for gastrointestinal endoscopists. Gastroenterol Hepatol. 2022;18(3):133.
6. Fujishiro M, Yahagi N, Kashimura K, Mizushima Y, Oka M, Enomoto S, et al. Comparison of various submucosal injection solutions for maintaining mucosal elevation during endoscopic mucosal resection. Endoscopy. 2004;36(7):579–83. Available from: https://pubmed.ncbi.nlm.nih.gov/15243878/
7. Bruno MJ. Magnification endoscopy, high resolution endoscopy, and chromoscopy; towards a better optical diagnosis. Gut. 2003;52(Suppl 4) Available from: https://pubmed.ncbi.nlm.nih.gov/12746262/:7iv.
8. Muto M, Horimatsu T, Ezoe Y, Morita S, Miyamoto S. Improving visualization techniques by narrow band imaging and magnification endoscopy. J Gastroenterol Hepatol. 2009;24(8):1333–46. Available from: https://pubmed.ncbi.nlm.nih.gov/19702901/
9. Liu L, Hofstetter WL, Rashid A, Swisher SG, Correa AM, Ajani JA, Hamilton SR, Wu TT. Significance of the depth of tumor invasion and lymph node metastasis in superficially invasive (T1) esophageal adenocarcinoma. Am J Surg Pathol. 2005;29(8):1079–85.
10. Westerterp M, Koppert LB, Buskens CJ, Tilanus HW, Ten Kate FJW, Bergman JJHGM, et al. Outcome of surgical treatment for early adenocarcinoma of the esophagus or gastro-esophageal junction. Virchows Arch. 2005;446(5):497–504. Available from: https://pubmed.ncbi.nlm.nih.gov/15838647/
11. Gotoda T, Yamamoto H, Soetikno RM. Endoscopic submucosal dissection of early gastric cancer. J Gastroenterol. 2006;41(10):929–42. Available from: https://pubmed.ncbi.nlm.nih.gov/17096062/

Chapter 3
Endoscopic Submucosal Dissection (ESD)

Kamil Erozkan and Emre Gorgun

Background

- Sporadic colorectal cancer arises from premalignant lesions, which can be surgically removed before the development of invasive carcinoma. Screening colonoscopy and subsequent polypectomy are widely acknowledged as effective measures in reducing the incidence of colorectal cancer and its associated mortality [1].
- Polyps smaller than 10 mm detected during colonoscopy screenings are typically excised with a cold snare. Larger polyps need historically segmental resections or advanced polypectomy techniques that were developed more recently. Surgical organ resections can lead to significant increase in mortality and morbidity, increased postoperative pain and blood loss, and prolonged length of hospital stay.
- Histopathology for such premalignant lesions after major surgeries often reveal a high percentage of benign nature [2], thus putting patients at unnecessary risk. Roughly 15% of colonic polyps necessitate advanced polypectomy techniques due to their size, location, or appearance [3]. Improvements in polypectomy techniques may help to minimize the need for surgical resection and decrease associated risks. Thereby, it prevents overtreatment and ensures complete resection.
- Advanced polypectomy techniques, such as endoscopic mucosal resection (EMR) and endoscopic submucosal dissection (ESD) or hybrid EMR–ESD procedures, have been proposed to remove large colorectal lesions.

K. Erozkan · E. Gorgun (✉)
Department of Colorectal Surgery, Digestive Disease and Surgery Institute, Cleveland Clinic, Cleveland, OH, USA
e-mail: erozkak@ccf.org; gorgune@ccf.org

M. Ujiki, Z. M. Callahan (eds.), *Third Space Endoscopy*,
https://doi.org/10.1007/978-3-031-84509-3_3

- ESD has gained popularity in Asia for removing upper gastrointestinal lesions [4]. In the early 2000s, the technique was also first described for colorectal lesions [5]. However, performing ESD in the colon and rectum presents technical difficulties due to the thickness of the colorectal wall, colonic folds, flexures, and peristalsis. Despite these challenges, the possibility of preventing colorectal cancer and the increasing demand in minimally invasive procedures have led to a growing interest in advanced polypectomy techniques for colorectal lesions. Moreover, ESD offers benefits such as shorter hospital stay, less postoperative pain, and lower mortality and morbidity rates compared to major surgery [6].
- Following successful initial studies and further research, ESD has been incorporated into guidelines for treating colorectal lesions. It is now a widely accepted approach for removing such lesions worldwide and gaining popularity in Western medical practices as well.
- This chapter provides an in-depth review of ESD, including its indications, technical steps, and outcomes.

Indications

General

- According to both Asian and Western guidelines, endoscopic submucosal dissection is advised for lesions larger than 20 mm and should be performed by an advanced endoscopist. The US Multi-Society Task Force on Colorectal Cancer recommends snare polypectomy for lesions smaller than 10 mm. EMR approach can be preferred for lesions between 10 and 20 mm.
- Although Asian-based guidelines have previously dominated the field, Western guidelines about ESD are growing now. Understanding both sets of guidelines can help clinicians make informed decisions regarding the use of ESD in patient care.

American Gastroenterology Association (AGA) Indications [7]

- Kudo V-type pit pattern.
- Depressed component (Paris 0–IIc).
- Complex morphology (0–Is or 0–IIa + Is).
- Rectosigmoid location.
- LST NG ≥20 mm.
- Granular LST ≥30 mm.
- Residual or recurrent colorectal adenomas.

Japan Gastroenterological Endoscopy Society (JGES) Recommendations [8]

- Lesions for which en bloc resection with snare EMR is challenging to apply.
  - LST-nongranular (LST-NG), particularly LST-NG pseudo-depressed type.
  - Lesions showing a Kudo type-V_I invasive pit pattern.
  - Carcinoma with submucosal infiltration.
  - Large depressed-type lesion.
  - Large, elevated lesion suspected to be a cancer.
- Mucosal lesions with submucosal fibrosis.
- Local residual early carcinoma after endoscopic resection.

Other Societal Recommendations

- European Society of Gastrointestinal Endoscopy (ESGE) recommendations are similar to the JGES guidelines [9].

Patient Evaluation

Initial Evaluation

- Before the procedure, it is crucial to obtain previous colonoscopy reports and carefully evaluate colored images of the colon and rectum to assess the lesion in detail. This will help the endoscopist determine if additional equipment may be necessary during the procedure.
- It is also crucial to obtain a detailed medical history from the patient, particularly focusing on anticoagulant use and dosage.

Diagnostic Studies

- Several preoperative applications can be used to ensure accurate diagnosis and successful treatment of colorectal lesions. Adequate bowel preparation is necessary to enable the identification of lesions during the initial colonoscopic examination. In cases where bowel preparation is inadequate, washing the lesion surface can be a good approach. Irrigation pumps can be used in low pressure setting for this purpose.

- Endoscopic evaluation of the polyp's appearance can aid in determining the likelihood of underlying malignancy. It is essential to evaluate lesions from all angles using proper inflation, deflation, and maneuvers. This assessment is crucial for effective preoperative management and treatment.
- Identifying the depth of invasion can be challenging. Magnifying chromoendoscopy and narrow-band imaging (NBI) can be used to assess the atypia in a tumor and the depth of invasion. The Japan Narrow-Band Imaging (NBI) Expert Team (JNET) classification, which subdivides lesions into types 1, 2A, 2B, and 3 according to surface morphology, is widely accepted for this purpose (Fig. 3.1). The types 1, 2A, 2B, and 3 describe hyperplastic lesions, low-grade dysplasia, high-grade dysplasia, and invasive carcinoma, respectively.
- Similarly, pit patterns can be used as a visual diagnostic tool. Kudo et al. initially introduced "pit patterns" using magnifying chromoendoscopy to classify lesions based on the surface morphology of crypt openings [10] (Fig. 3.2). According to this classification, type III_S, III_L, and IV lesions strongly indicate adenomatous lesions, whereas type V_I and V_N are associated with early colorectal cancer.
- In Paris classification, height of lesions is also evaluated in addition to surface morphology (Fig. 3.3a). A different subclassification is used for laterally spreading tumors (LST), which are larger, flat, and/or sessile lesions ≥10 mm. LSTs have separate molecular pathways associated with submucosal invasion and fibrosis risk. Morphological classification of LST and their correspondence with the Paris classification can be seen in Fig. 3.3b.
- Multimodal endoscopic examination is superior to the other imaging methods, such as computerized tomography or magnetic resonance imaging, for detecting premalignant lesions and early cancer [11].
- A biopsy is not recommended due to the possibility of creating submucosal fibrosis and inappropriate sampling from the suspicious lesion [12].
- In suspicious cases, the possible invasion depth of colorectal polyps can be evaluated using a high-frequency mini-probe ultrasound inserted through the scope's working channel. This assessment helps to determine whether there is an invasion of the muscularis propria [7].

Preoperative Preparation

- Depending on the patient's medication regimen, anticoagulants may need to be stopped for 2–7 days before the procedure.
- ESD can be performed in either endoscopy suites or operating rooms, but the operating rooms may be preferred for patients with comorbidities or high-risk lesions. Additionally, procedures can turn into combined endo-laparoscopies in cases of perforation or when a full-thickness resection is necessary (Fig. 3.4).

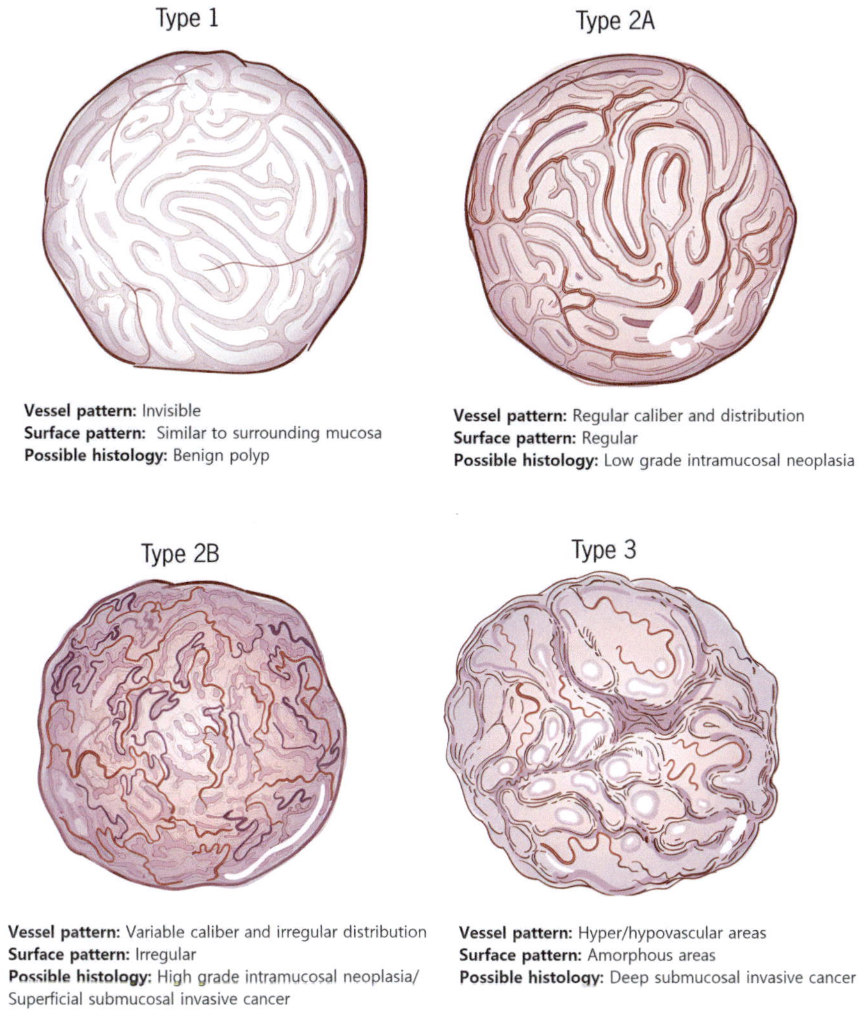

Fig. 3.1 JNET classification

Technique

Planning

- Before the beginning of the procedure in the operating room, general endotracheal anesthesia is our routine preference with endotracheal intubation in case of a need for laparoscopy. Carbon dioxide (CO_2) should be used as the insufflating gas during the colonoscopy.

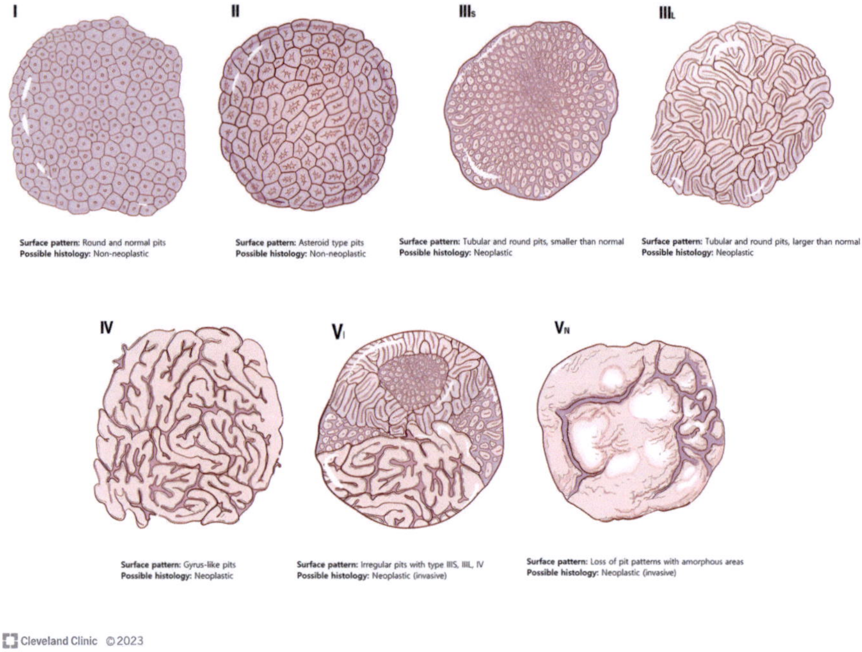

Fig. 3.2 Kudo's pit pattern classification

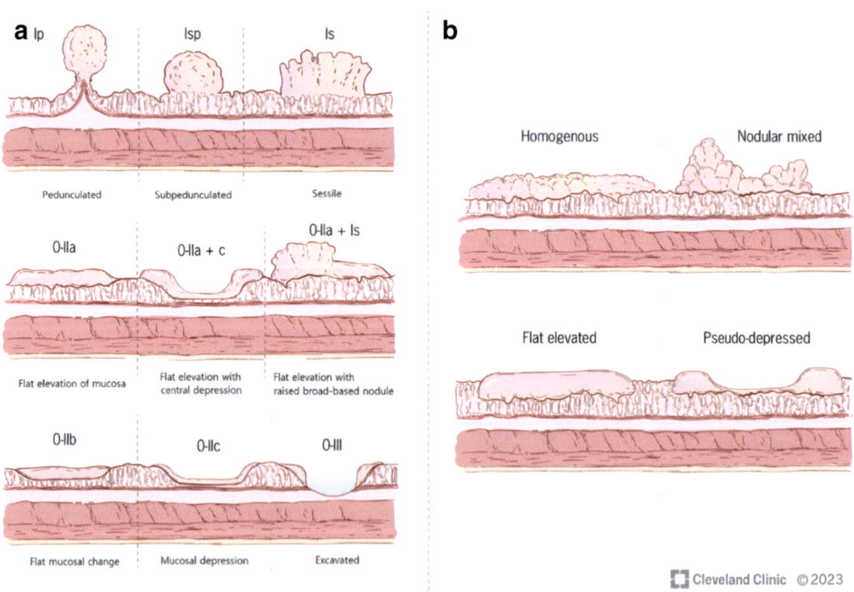

Fig. 3.3 (**a**) Paris classification. (**b**) Subtypes of laterally spreading tumors

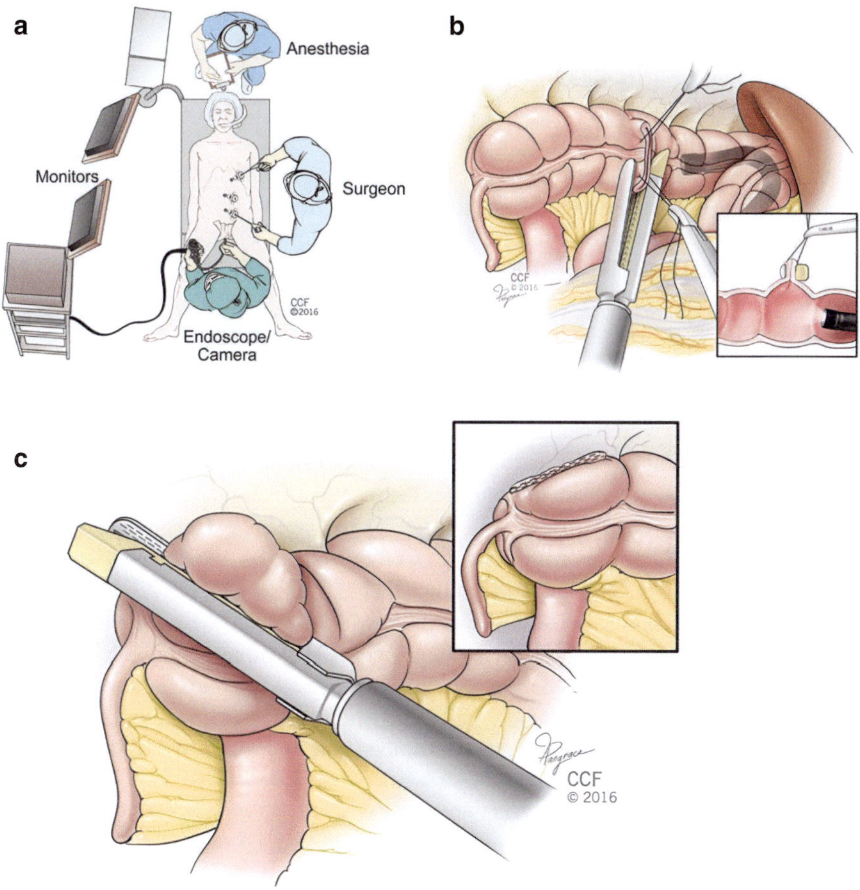

Fig. 3.4 Combined endo-laparoscopic ESD. (**a**) Operating room setup for combined endo-laparoscopic ESD. (**b**) Stapler can be used to complete full-thickness combined endo-laparoscopic ESD for lesions not amenable for endoscopic resection, and simultaneous scoping can be used to assess the passage and ensure that lumen is not occluded during/after resection. (**c**) For lesions located on difficult locations such as cecum, wedge resection can be performed to remove the lesion

- Colloid solution and an inert dye are two common elements of injection solution. Mixing small amounts of indigo carmine or methylene blue dye for the injection solution provides better visuals of the structures and vasculature. Several injectable solutions are available in ESD, including glycerol, diluted adrenaline (1 mL of 0.1% adrenalin), hyaluronic acid, and sterile saline. Normal saline disperses quickly and lasts only 1–10 minutes, while diluted hydroxypropyl methylcellulose (hypromellose) can be a cost-effective and prolonged alternative.
- Various FDA-approved solutions are available for lifting during local anal procedures, including LiftUp® (Ovesco Endoscopy AG, Tübingen, Germany), Blue

Eye™ (The Standard Co., Ltd., Gunpo-si, Korea), Blue Beacon™ (Micro-Tech Co., Ltd., Nanjing, China), EverLift™ Submucosal Lifting Agent (Gi Supply, Inc.), Eleview® (SIC 8000) (Cosmo Technologies, Ltd., Dublin, Ireland), and EndoClot® solution (EndoClot Plus Co., Ltd., Santa Clara, CA, USA). No mixing is required before injecting these premade solutions. Premixed solutions remain in the submucosal plane for long durations, reducing the procedure time by eliminating preparation steps and repeat injections.

- Choosing the appropriate needle size and injection technique can help ensure that the injectate is delivered accurately and efficiently, improving the safety and effectiveness of the ESD procedure. A 21- to 25-gauge injection needle catheter is typically used when delivering injectates during an ESD procedure. However, a larger bore needle may be required when dealing with viscous injectates. In some cases, ESD knives may have an integrated water jet channel within the device catheter, which can be used to deliver injectates.
- Multiple different types of endoknife combinations and instruments may be used during the procedure, including FlexKnife Electrosurgical Knife (Olympus, Tokyo, Japan), DualKnife™ (Olympus America Inc., Center Valley, PA), HookKnife™ (Olympus America Inc., Center Valley, PA), ITknife nano™ electrosurgical knife (Olympus America Inc., Center Valley, PA), ORISE ProKnife™ electrosurgical knife (Boston Scientific, Marlborough, MA), HybridKnife® (ERBE, Tübingen, Germany), and Coagrasper™ (Olympus America Inc., Center Valley, PA) (Fig. 3.5). A snare tip can also be used as an endoscopic knife.
- The DualKnife™ electrosurgical knife is a single-use instrument with an adjustable two-step knife length and a dome-shaped cutting section, making it easier to mark and incise in all directions.
- The HookKnife™ is a distal L-shaped hook with a rotational function that allows precise incision and dissection in longitudinal and lateral directions.
- The ITknife nano™ electrosurgical knife is a single-use device designed for precise and safe dissection in narrow lumens with a small, insulated tip, a proximally placed electrode, and a shorter knife length.

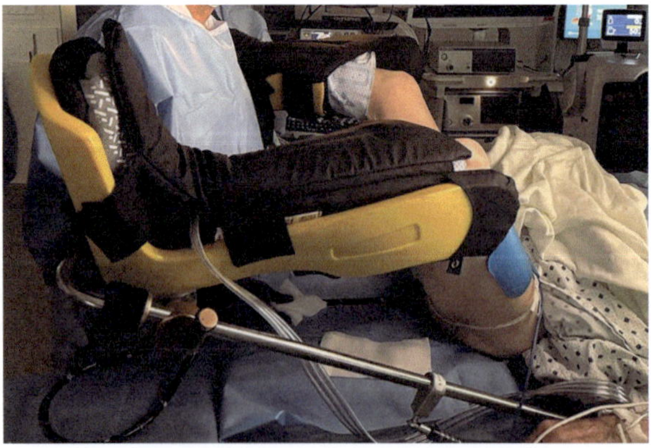

Fig. 3.5 Room setup and patient position for ESD

- ORISE ProKnife™ electrosurgical knife has a T-shaped electrode that can be used for injection simultaneously. It's designed to create a sustained lift without a device exchange for ESD procedures.
- The HybridKnife® is a single instrument that injects solution and facilitates dissection simultaneously. It is advantageous because both injection and dissection components can be introduced through the same channel, making it easier to maintain the location and avoid unnecessary withdrawal of the endoscope and instrument changes.
- The Coagrasper™ provides precise and adequate hemostasis by grasping a bleeding point or visible vessel and coagulating it.
- Using the proper coagulation devices and generators are essential, especially for endoluminal procedures. The most utilized energy towers are VIO®3 (Erbe USA, Inc., Marietta, GA, USA) and Geradores THUNDERBEAT (ESG-400 e USG-400) (Olympus America Inc., Center Valley, PA, USA). These generators are designed for endoluminal procedures providing different energy modalities, including swift, forced, and spray coagulation options. In their cutting mode, blended energy can be applied, combined with cutting and a blend of coagulation periods. Additionally, more coagulation can be added for patient-specific bleeding tendencies to minimize bleeding even in the cutting or blend mode. The other advantage of these generators is that in the blend cutting mode, application of pulsatile energy is enabled, which allows physicians to make a clear cut at superficial levels that can expose deeper vessels more clearly.
- ERBEJET® 2 (ERBE, Tübingen, Germany) is a water jet system that uses pressured saline injections instead of electrocautery or ultrasonic power. It allows for layer-specific procedures and simplified elevation in difficult anatomy. It is a recent development and may shorten dissection time and reduce perforation risk.

Endoscopic Access and Anatomical Landmarks

- The patient should be positioned in the modified lithotomy position with appropriate padding, leaving the leg extension portion of the surgical table in place to maintain a stable counter space during the procedure (Fig. 3.6). The operator should stand between the patient's legs for optimal access to the anus.
- The polyp should be identified and located, with efforts made to maneuver the colonoscope to position the polyp at the 6 o'clock position (Fig. 3.7). Specific position changes may be necessary for lesions in particular locations, such as the ileocecal valve. An upper or pediatric endoscopes should be selectively used based on the lesion's location and features.

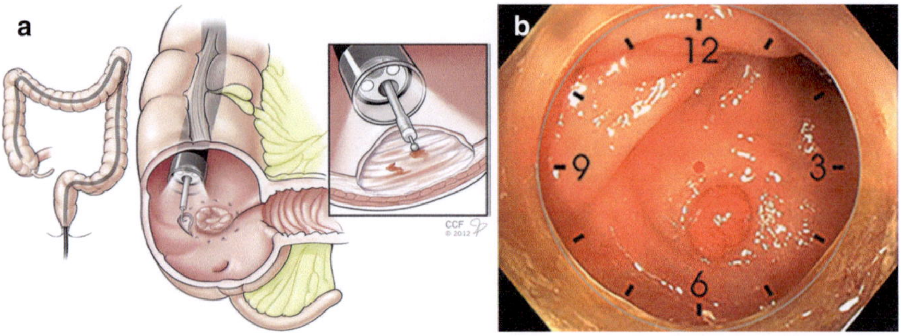

Fig. 3.6 Orientation and polyp position for ESD. (**a**) Orientation. (**b**) The lesion should be brought to the 6 o'clock position

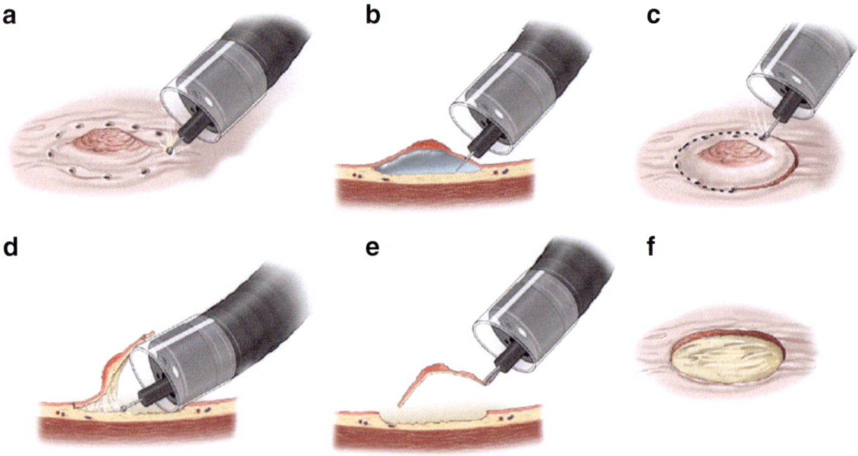

Fig. 3.7 Technical steps of ESD. (**a**) Marking. (**b**) Submucosal injection. (**c**) Incision. (**d**) Submucosal dissection. (**e**) Specimen extraction. (**f**) Resection bed

Marking and Mucosal Lift

- Mark the mucosa outside of the lesion with a 2–3 mm normal mucosal margin to help visualize the borders during ESD (Fig. 3.8). This step may not be necessary and can be skipped with increased experience.
- Lift the lesion with injectate to form a dissection plane between the mucosa and muscularis propria. Adequate lifting reduces the risk of perforation and transmural thermal injury by separating the lesion from the deeper muscularis propria layer and decreasing tissue resistance within the dissection plane.
- Inject the solution around the lesion to provide a margin of safety when incising the mucosa. As the dissection continues, the submucosal injection can be repeated periodically to expand the submucosal plane. Inject the solution on the far edge

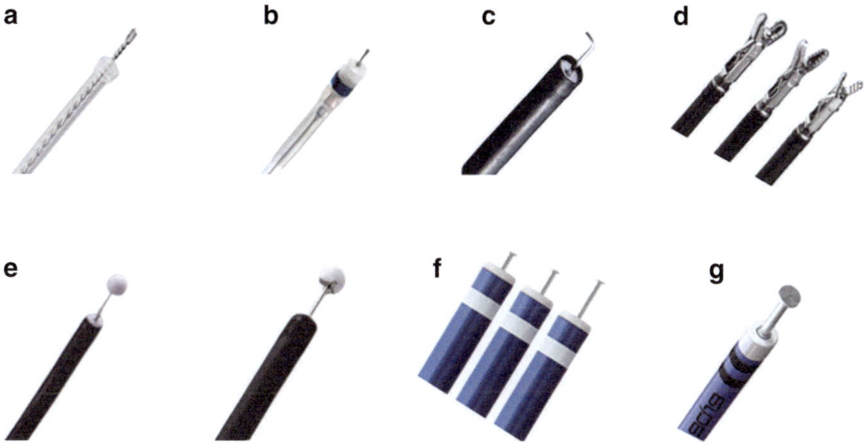

Fig. 3.8 Endoknife examples. (**a**) FlexKnife Electrosurgical Knife (Olympus, Tokyo, Japan), (**b**) DualKnife™ (Olympus America Inc., Center Valley, PA), (**c**) HookKnife™ (Olympus America Inc., Center Valley, PA), (**d**) Coagrasper™ (Olympus America Inc., Center Valley, PA), (**e**) The ITknife nano™ 1 and 2 electrosurgical knife (Olympus America Inc., Center Valley, PA), (**f**) ORISE ProKnife™ electrosurgical knife (Boston Scientific, Marlborough, MA), (**g**) HybridKnife® (ERBE, Tübingen, Germany)

of the lesion to ensure a clear view of the polyp located on a fold. This prevents the lesion from remaining behind the fold. The injection needle should be advanced tangentially to the mucosa. This way, deep or superficial injections can be prevented.

- Create the submucosal cushion by advancing the needle tip into the mucosa while the assisting physician starts the injection. The immediate elevation of the mucosa confirms entry into the correct plane. Ensure the injection material is evenly distributed in the submucosa to form adequate planes and facilitates safe dissection. If the lesion does not lift or there is extravasation of intraluminal fluid during injection, the needle can be gently advanced or withdrawn until the correct plane is identified.
- The "non-lifting sign" may indicate the presence of invasive disease or submucosal fibrosis. Stop the procedure when a deep invasion is suspected. However, it is possible to proceed in cases where non-lifting is from previous attempts at tissue resection. In cases where submucosal fibrosis is suspected, the incision should be started further from the lesion. This will facilitate entry into the submucosal space where normal tissue is located.

Mucosal Incision and Dissection

- After the submucosal injection, perform a partial circumferential incision starting from the distal border of the lesion. In some cases, retroflexion may be needed for an adequate incision. A complete circumferential incision can increase fluid leakage and make subsequent lifts more difficult.
- After the initial incision, continue the submucosal dissection, deepening as needed until the lesion is fully separated from the underlying submucosa. Dissection proceeds tangentially (parallel) to the submucosa in the direction of the identified muscularis propria. Repeat this process until dissection is complete. Resect the lesion en bloc following complete dissection.
- Ensure the dissection plane is maintained during the procedure to avoid perforation or bleeding. Stay within the established plane.

Adjuncts to Dissection

- Aid visualization by attaching a clear cap distally to elevate the overlying mucosa and create traction. Changing the patient's position to use gravity can also improve exposure in bleeding or difficultly located polyps.
- Clips and rubber bands can be used for traction (Fig. 3.9). Alternatively, transanal flexible traction graspers are excellent options for traction in distal lesions (Fig. 3.10).
- Balloon inflation over the scope can stabilize the lumen, and a balloon overtube can be used for standard ESD when dissection is challenging due to paradoxical movements. After reaching the lesion, the balloon overtube can be fixed with the balloon attached to the distal end (Fig. 3.11).

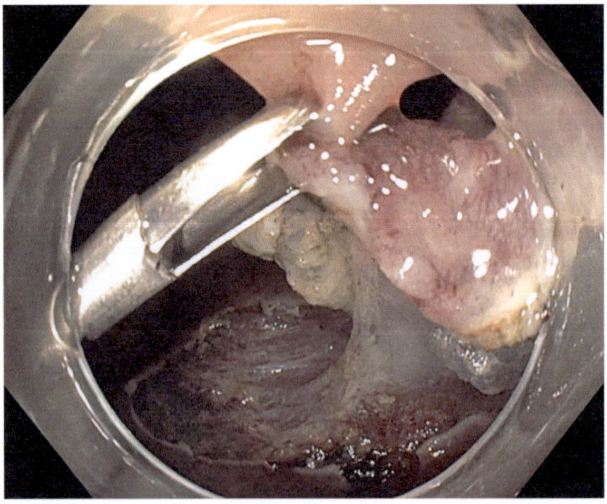

Fig. 3.9 "Gorgun" clip and lift technique during ESD

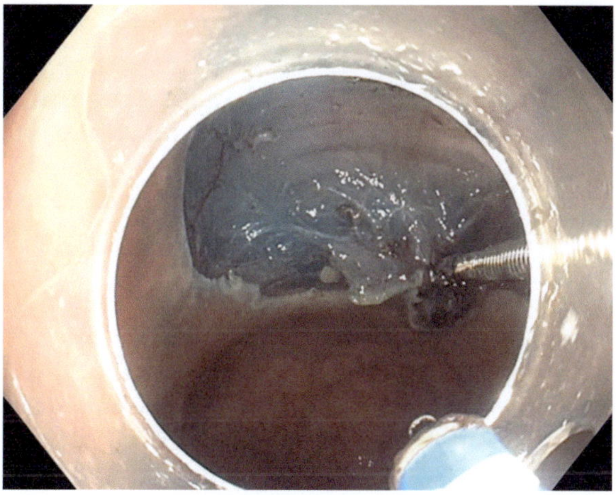

Fig. 3.10 External traction with grasping device

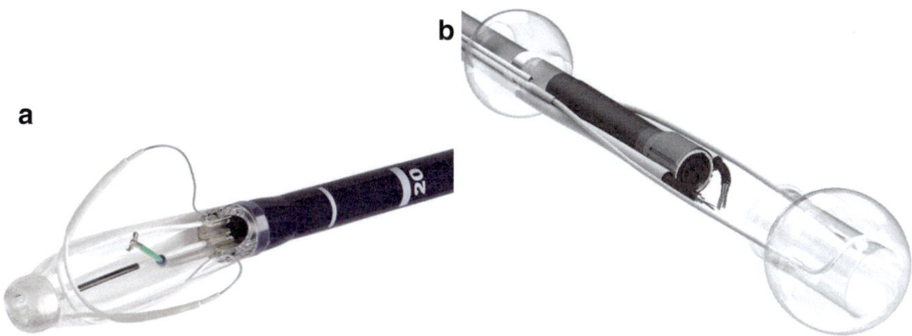

Fig. 3.11 Endoscopic surgical platform examples. (**a**) The ORISE TRS platform by Boston Scientific (Marlborough, MA) has a stabilization cage with two available retractors to provide counter tension. (**b**) The DiLumen C2 platform by Lumendi (Westport, CT) has a fore and aft balloon to straighten and stabile the colon with two available terratros to create tension

- Balloon-assisted retraction is another advantage of this method. After initial incision and appreciating the submucosa, an endoclip can be applied to the side of the lesion and the balloon. This method provides a stable environment for the endoscopist and allows for the continuous exposure of the submucosal layer.
- Another trick for improving stability is the J maneuver (retroflexed scope). Particularly in the right colon, the J maneuver makes the endoscopic submucosal dissection technically feasible.

Specimen Removal and Hemostasis

- The resected lesion is placed in a net and removed from the patient. The specimen should be stretched onto a board with pins before sending it for histopathological analysis (Fig. 3.12).
- The resection bed should be examined routinely for any complications after the resection. Submucosal defects or bleeding can be observed due to thermal injury or minimal trauma.
- Minor defects can be repaired with endoscopic sutures or clips, which may help prevent delayed perforation and bleeding (Fig. 3.13). Over-the-scope clips are used for large perforations. For larger defects, surgical operations may be needed.
- Minimal bleeding may occur during the procedure and should not be alarming. Visible vessels can be cauterized to reduce the risk of bleeding. Endoscopic clips and snare coagulation can be used to control bleeding.

Postoperative Care

- Endoscopists should monitor patients for signs of bleeding or perforation and take appropriate action if necessary.
- Patients undergoing ESD are typically observed 3–4 h after the procedure, and those with complicated or larger lesions may stay overnight. Overnight observation is strongly recommended to recognize any potential early procedure-related complications.
- Abdominal X-rays may be used to check for the presence of free air after a difficult ESD procedure.
- Prophylactic antibiotics are unnecessary, and no dietary restrictions are required after the procedure.
- The aim of follow-up colonoscopy and surveillance after ESD is early detection of local recurrences and/or metachronous lesions. Currently, there is no consen-

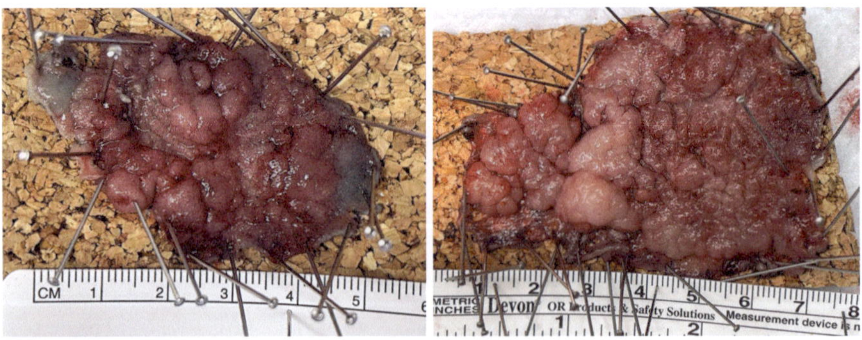

Fig. 3.12 Specimen examples

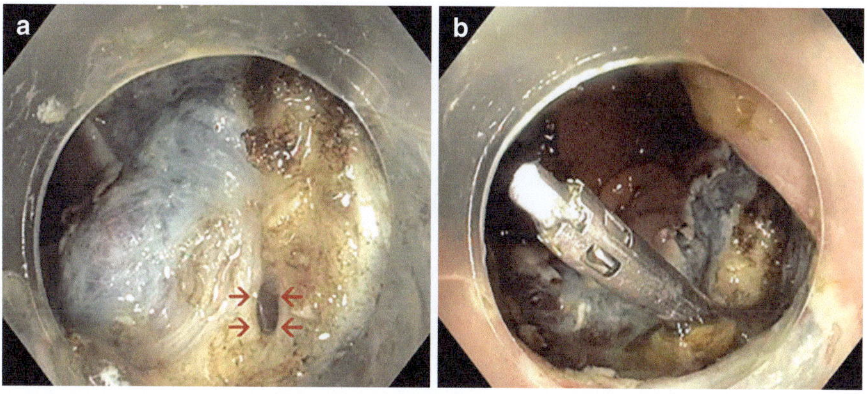

Fig. 3.13 Endoscopic clip placement for closure after full-thickness perforation. (**a**) Muscularis propria defect. (**b**) Closure with clip

sus on surveillance after mucosal resection. A repeat colonoscopy after 6 months is recommended to confirm complete polyp removal and the absence of recurrent adenomatous tissue. The next colonoscopy should be in the first and third years of the operation.
- The pathologic characteristics and quality of the resected specimen determine the proposed surveillance and individual risk factors, including more than one lesion, previous carcinoma history, and accompanying comorbidities.

Outcomes

- Endoscopic resection can be applied successfully in 92% of cases [2]. En bloc resection rates are between 83% and 97% [13–17].
- ESD is associated with a lower complication rate and has favorable en bloc and curative resection rates for early cancers with low risk of lymph node metastasis [18]. In early cancer patients, the en bloc and curative resection rates with ESD are 87% and 80%, respectively. The 3-year overall survival rate exceeded 99% for ESD procedures.
- Endoscopic methods at the resection site carry the potential for recurrence, with local recurrence after ESD being approximately 1% for superficial lesions [13–17].
- According to the Japanese Society for Cancer of the Colon and Rectum, lymph node harvest and surgical resection are necessary for cancer patients in cases of R1 resection, vascular or lymphatic invasion, tumor budding or depth of invasion greater than 1000 mm, and poorly differentiated adenocarcinoma after the histopathological examination [18].
- ESD is more cost-effective than major surgeries and provides advantages such as less postoperative pain, shorter hospital stays, and increased quality of life with

early ambulation and organ preservation. It also leads to better functional outcomes [19].

- Institutions with lower total case numbers have reported higher complication rates in endoscopic resections [20]. The most common complications are perforation and bleeding, which can occur during or after the procedure. Perforation rates are associated with increased tumor size and fibrosis and are reported to be between 2.5% and 18% of all patients [21–25]. Immediate perforation rates are higher than delayed perforation rates, with the latter being less than 0.5%. Due to the risk of fecal residue leakage and peritonitis, surgical treatment may be necessary in cases with suspicion of delayed perforation. Perforation of malignant lesions during ESD can result in potential tumor seeding, as evidenced by the more robust gastric cancer literature.
- Studies have reported bleeding rates ranging from 2% to 13% [22, 24]. Delayed bleeding rates have been reported to be 2% [15], and these may require exploration and resections if they cannot be controlled endoscopically. Workup includes serial CBC checks and close monitoring. Blood transfusion is given only when indicated, and patients are scoped in the endoscopy unit if bleeding is continuous. In our experience, most bleeding is self-limited and is more common in patients with chronic anticoagulation use.
- Post-ESD electrocoagulation syndrome can be seen in up to 40% of patients. Patients have abdominal pain, fever, and disturbances in bowel habits without a sign of perforation. It's often managed nonoperatively. General risk factors include right colonic procedures, prolonged procedure times, and large lesions greater than 40 mm. Complaints of pain can be common after ESD. Unremitting pain may warrant advanced radiologic assessment, especially if accompanying symptoms are present.
- Strictures can develop in large lesions, lesions with long longitudinal lengths, and lesions with mucosal defects greater than three-quarters of the luminal circumference. However, stricture has only been reported for several rectal lesions (Fig. 3.14).
- Abscess development is often caused by delayed perforation after local anal procedures. Other rare complications include urinary retention, diarrhea, ileus, splenic injury, mesenteric hemorrhage, diverticulitis, appendicitis, and pancreatitis.

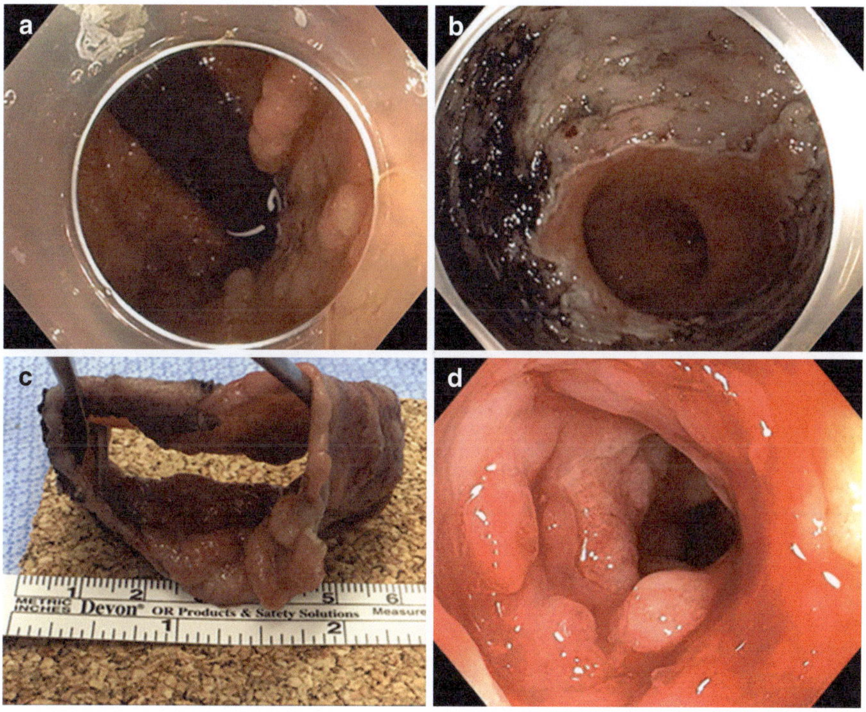

Fig. 3.14 Stricture development and treatment. (**a**) Circumferential lesion. (**b**) Resection bed. (**c**) Specimen. (**d**) Stricture

Pearls	Pitfalls
Overtreatment	Advanced polypectomy techniques are preferred over major colorectal resections for benign polyps and early-stage colorectal cancers For palliative management, it is a viable option for patients unsuitable for oncological resection due to their general condition, age, or other factors Surgeons should choose the most appropriate technique based on the polyp's size, location, and morphology. Complex cases should be managed with a multidisciplinary team In rectal cancer patients with a complete clinical response following total neoadjuvant treatment, selective ESD use can expand the organ preservation opportunity
Experience	Good colonoscopy skills and a minimum of 200–300 colonoscopies per year are necessary to start ESD training Attending didactic and hands-on ESD courses before scheduling initial ESD cases is strongly recommended The learning curve for ESD has not been widely investigated, but ESD competency was reported to be 20–200 cases Start with small and easily accessible lesions to gain experience. Obtain informed consent for the procedure and possible complications Informed consent should be obtained for possible laparoscopic assistance and bowel resection if ESD cannot be completed

(continued)

Pearls	Pitfalls
Preoperative planning	Perform a full colonoscopy in case of possible synchronized lesions Use advanced imaging techniques to determine the potential malignancy of the lesion
Non-lifting	Use the appropriate lifting technique based on the location and characteristics of the lesion. Avoid over-dissection of the submucosal plane to prevent perforation The "non-lifting sign" may indicate the presence of invasive disease or submucosal fibrosis. Stop the procedure when deep invasion is suspected. However, it is possible to proceed in cases where non-lifting is from previous attempts at tissue resection
Invasive carcinoma	In the case of early malignancy, microscopic examination of endoscopically resected specimens is particularly important because a precise histopathological analysis influences the potential need for further surgery Patients with non-curative ESD resections should be referred to surgery
Traction	A clear cap is commonly utilized to provide traction. However, in cases where traction is insufficient, alternative methods such as clips, rubber bands, and external flexible graspers can be employed to improve traction Balloon-assisted endoscopy also provides traction. Moreover, this technique enhances stability when dissection is challenging due to paradoxical movements
Perforation	Dissection should proceed tangentially (parallel) to the submucosa in the direction of the identified muscularis propria to minimize the risk of complications, such as perforation or bleeding during the procedure Perforations should be immediately closed using endoclips or endoscopic suture techniques to prevent further complications
Bleeding	Any bleeding that occurs during the resection should be promptly managed by coagulation. Endoclips may also be utilized to control bleeding during the procedure Cleaning the resection field is important, as it will allow the endoscopist to detect any bleeding immediately and intervene
Delayed complications	It should be kept in mind that post-procedural abdominal pain, tachycardia, hypotension, and physical examination findings may be important It is conducted overnight to detect any potential delayed complications that may arise after the procedure is highly recommended
Stricture	After the excision of large lesions, strictures can develop in the long term. Therefore, close endoscopic follow-up should be considered to detect and manage them promptly

References

1. Zauber AG, Winawer SJ, O'Brien MJ, Lansdorp-Vogelaar I, van Ballegooijen M, Hankey BF, et al. Colonoscopic polypectomy and long-term prevention of colorectal-cancer deaths. N Engl J Med. 2012;366(8):687–96. Available from: https://www.nejm.org/doi/full/10.1056/NEJMoa1100370
2. Gorgun E, Benlice C, Abbas MA, Steele S. Experience in colon sparing surgery in North America: advanced endoscopic approaches for complex colorectal lesions. Surg Endosc. 2018;32(7):3114–21. Available from: https://pubmed.ncbi.nlm.nih.gov/29362906/

3. Zhang M, Shin EJ. Successful endoscopic strategies for difficult polypectomy. Curr Opin Gastroenterol. 2013;29(5):489–94. Available from: https://pubmed.ncbi.nlm.nih.gov/23921466/
4. Saito Y, Sakamoto T, Nakajima T, Matsuda T. Colorectal ESD: current indications and latest technical advances. Gastrointest Endosc Clin N Am. 2014;24(2):245–55. Available from: https://pubmed.ncbi.nlm.nih.gov/24679235/
5. Yamamoto H, Kawata H, Sunada K, Sasaki A, Nakazawa K, Miyata T, et al. Successful en-bloc resection of large superficial tumors in the stomach and colon using sodium hyaluronate and small-caliber-tip transparent hood. Endoscopy. 2003;35(8):690–4. Available from: https://pubmed.ncbi.nlm.nih.gov/12929067/
6. Gamaleldin M, Benlice C, Delaney CP, Steele S, Gorgun E. Management of the colorectal polyp referred for resection: a case-matched comparison of advanced endoscopic surgery and laparoscopic colectomy. Surgery. 2018;163(3):522–7. Available from: https://pubmed.ncbi.nlm.nih.gov/29361367/
7. Draganov PV, Wang AY, Othman MO, Fukami N. AGA Institute clinical practice update: endoscopic submucosal dissection in the United States. Clin Gastroenterol Hepatol. 2019;17(1):16–25. Available from: https://pubmed.ncbi.nlm.nih.gov/30077787/
8. Tanaka S, Kashida H, Saito Y, Yahagi N, Yamano H, Saito S, et al. JGES guidelines for colorectal endoscopic submucosal dissection/endoscopic mucosal resection. Dig Endosc. 2015;27(4):417–34. Available from: https://pubmed.ncbi.nlm.nih.gov/25652022/
9. Pimentel-Nunes P, Dinis-Ribeiro M, Ponchon T, Repici A, Vieth M, De Ceglie A, et al. Endoscopic submucosal dissection: European Society of Gastrointestinal Endoscopy (ESGE) guideline. Endoscopy. 2015;47(9):829–54. Available from: https://pubmed.ncbi.nlm.nih.gov/26317585/
10. Kudo SE, Tamura S, Nakajima T, Yamano HO, Kusaka H, Watanabe H. Diagnosis of colorectal tumorous lesions by magnifying endoscopy. Gastrointest Endosc. 1996;44(1):8–14. Available from: https://pubmed.ncbi.nlm.nih.gov/8836710/
11. Emmanuel A, Lapa C, Ghosh A, Gulati S, Burt M, Hayee B, et al. Multimodal endoscopic assessment guides treatment decisions for rectal early neoplastic tumors. Dis Colon Rectum. 2020;63(3):326–35. Available from: https://pubmed.ncbi.nlm.nih.gov/32045398/
12. Pouw RE, Bisschops R, Gecse KB, De Hertogh G, Iacucci M, Rutter M, et al. Endoscopic tissue sampling – part 2: lower gastrointestinal tract. European Society of Gastrointestinal Endoscopy (ESGE) guideline. Endoscopy. 2021;53(12):1261–73. Available from: https://pubmed.ncbi.nlm.nih.gov/34715702/
13. Lee EJ, Lee JB, Lee SH, Kim DS, Lee DH, Lee DS, et al. Endoscopic submucosal dissection for colorectal tumors – 1,000 colorectal ESD cases: one specialized institute's experiences. Surg Endosc. 2013;27(1):31–9. Available from: https://pubmed.ncbi.nlm.nih.gov/22729707/
14. Oka S, Tanaka S, Saito Y, Iishi H, Kudo SE, Ikematsu H, et al. Local recurrence after endoscopic resection for large colorectal neoplasia: a multicenter prospective study in Japan. Am J Gastroenterol. 2015;110(5):697–707. Available from: https://pubmed.ncbi.nlm.nih.gov/25848926/
15. Repici A, Hassan C, De Paula PD, Pagano N, Arezzo A, Zullo A, et al. Efficacy and safety of endoscopic submucosal dissection for colorectal neoplasia: a systematic review. Endoscopy. 2012;44(2):137–50. Available from: https://pubmed.ncbi.nlm.nih.gov/22271024/
16. Repici A, Pellicano R, Strangio G, Danese S, Fagoonee S, Malesci A. Endoscopic mucosal resection for early colorectal neoplasia: pathologic basis, procedures, and outcomes. Dis Colon Rectum. 2009;52(8):1502–15. Available from: https://pubmed.ncbi.nlm.nih.gov/19617768/
17. Tanaka S, Terasaki M, Kanao H, Oka S, Chayama K. Current status and future perspectives of endoscopic submucosal dissection for colorectal tumors. Dig Endosc. 2012;24(Suppl 1):73–9. Available from: https://pubmed.ncbi.nlm.nih.gov/22533757/
18. Hashiguchi Y, Muro K, Saito Y, Ito Y, Ajioka Y, Hamaguchi T, et al. Japanese Society for cancer of the colon and Rectum (JSCCR) guidelines 2019 for the treatment of colorectal cancer. Int J Clin Oncol. 2020;25(1):1–42. Available from: https://pubmed.ncbi.nlm.nih.gov/31203527/

19. Nakamura F, Saito Y, Haruyama S, Sekiguchi M, Yamada M, Sakamoto T, et al. Short-term prospective questionnaire study of early postoperative quality of life after colorectal endoscopic submucosal dissection. Dig Dis Sci. 2017;62(12):3325–35. Available from: https://pubmed.ncbi.nlm.nih.gov/29043596/
20. Saito Y, Uraoka T, Yamaguchi Y, Hotta K, Sakamoto N, Ikematsu H, et al. A prospective, multicenter study of 1111 colorectal endoscopic submucosal dissections (with video). Gastrointest Endosc. 2010;72(6):1217–25. Available from: https://pubmed.ncbi.nlm.nih.gov/21030017/
21. Akintoye E, Kumar N, Aihara H, Nas H, Thompson C. Colorectal endoscopic submucosal dissection: a systematic review and meta-analysis. Endosc Int Open. 2016;4(10):E1030–44. Available from: https://pubmed.ncbi.nlm.nih.gov/27747275/
22. Rahmi G, Hotayt B, Chaussade S, Lepilliez V, Giovannini M, Coumaros D, et al. Endoscopic submucosal dissection for superficial rectal tumors: prospective evaluation in France. Endoscopy. 2014;46(8):670–6. Available from: https://pubmed.ncbi.nlm.nih.gov/24977400/
23. Saito Y, Fukuzawa M, Matsuda T, Fukunaga S, Sakamoto T, Uraoka T, et al. Clinical outcome of endoscopic submucosal dissection versus endoscopic mucosal resection of large colorectal tumors as determined by curative resection. Surg Endosc. 2010;24(2):343–52. Available from: https://pubmed.ncbi.nlm.nih.gov/19517168/
24. Sakamoto T, Mori G, Yamada M, Kinjo Y, So E, Abe S, et al. Endoscopic submucosal dissection for colorectal neoplasms: a review. World J Gastroenterol. 2014;20(43):16153.
25. Takamaru H, Saito Y, Yamada M, Tsuruki ES, Kinjo Y, Otake Y, et al. Clinical impact of endoscopic clip closure of perforations during endoscopic submucosal dissection for colorectal tumors. Gastrointest Endosc. 2016;84(3):494–502.e1. Available from: https://pubmed.ncbi.nlm.nih.gov/26774353/

Chapter 4
Endoscopic Full-Thickness Resection (EFTR)

Jamie Benson, Joshua Lyons, and Jeffrey Marks

Background

- Resection of neoplasia involving the mucosa and submucosal layers has been facilitated using endoscopic mucosal resection (EMR) and endoscopic submucosal dissection (ESD). Obtaining R0 resection in difficult to remove lesions and neoplasms that involve the muscularis propria led to the emergence of endoscopic full-thickness resection (EFTR).
- The first EFTR prototype was created in 2001 but was only used in animal models [1]. The progression of endoscopic closure techniques for luminal defects following EFTR led to improved clinical outcomes and the safe closure of larger defects.
- Initially, endoscopic luminal defect closure consisted of through-the-scope (TTS) clips, which had limitations on luminal defect size and the lack of full-thickness approximation. An endoloop clip-assisted method improved the closure of larger defects however still possessed the lack of full-thickness approximation. Further improvements in EFTR defect closure occurred with the introduction of over-the-scope-clips (OTSC) for the closure of GI perforations, fistulas, and hemostasis [2]. The first clinical case of EFTR using OTSC occurred in 2014 [3], and since then, many studies have been reported.
- An additional technique that involves the flexible endoscopic suturing device (OverStitch endoscopic suturing system, Apollo Endosurgery, Austin, Texas, USA) allows closure of larger defects with the addition of full-thickness approximation.

J. Benson · J. Lyons · J. Marks (✉)
Department of Surgery, University Hospitals Cleveland Medical Center, Cleveland, OH, USA
e-mail: Jamie.Benson@uhhospitals.org; Jeffrey.Marks@uhhospitals.org

M. Ujiki, Z. M. Callahan (eds.), *Third Space Endoscopy*,
https://doi.org/10.1007/978-3-031-84509-3_4

Indications

- In the upper gastrointestinal tract, EFTR is indicated for subepithelial tumors (SETs) including symptomatic lesions (which typically involve pain, obstructive symptoms, or bleeding), neuroendocrine tumors, adenomas in transmural scars, mesenchymal tumors (e.g., GIST, Schwannoma, leiomyoma) that are >2 cm in size or have high-risk EUS features, or if the tumor has significant muscularis propria involvement or an extra-luminal component.
- In colorectal surgery, EFTR is indicated in non-lifting and/or residual lesions after failed ESD, adenomas near the appendix/diverticulum not amenable to EMR/ESD, or early carcinoma [4, 5].

Patient Evaluation

Initial Evaluation

- A thorough medical history and physical examination is taken to assess the patient's general health and identify any potential contraindications to the procedure.
- A multidisciplinary team, including a gastroenterologist, surgeon, and pathologist, should be involved in the preoperative planning.

Diagnostic Studies

- Imaging studies, such as computed tomography (CT) or magnetic resonance imaging (MRI), can be performed to evaluate the size, location, and depth of the lesion, as well as possible exophytic nature making endoscopic resection more difficult or contraindicated.
- Before EFTR, the lesion must be carefully evaluated using endoscopy, including endoscopic ultrasound (EUS), to determine the depth of invasion and whether the lesion can be completely removed endoscopically. The lesion should be well-defined and located in a surgically accessible area.

Technique

Planning

- Equipment commonly used for EFTR are as follows: single-channel gastroscope for resection (GIF HQ 190, Olympus, MA, USA) and dual-channel endoscope for suturing (CF 2T160L, Olympus, MA, USA), electrosurgical knife (e.g., ITknife™, DualKnife™, Hooknife™, Olympus, MA, USA; HybridKnife®, ERBE, MA, USA), electrosurgical generator unit, CO_2 insufflator, injection needle, TTS clips and OTSC, and endoscopic suturing system (OverStitch™, Apollo Endosurgery, TX, USA).

Tunneled Exposed EFTR

- In tunneled exposed EFTR, which is essentially submucosal tunnel endoscopic resection (STER), a mucosal incision is made followed by tunneling to allow access to a submucosal lesion, which is resected and removed prior to closure of the tunnel entry site. STER is typically used for SETs but not for mucosal neoplasia. Due to the small tunnel size, STER has the most practical success for lesions ≤4 cm in diameter [6].
- Full-thickness closure is not required. Closure of only the mucosal defect is necessary to maintain luminal integrity. Standard TTS clips have been used for closure of the mucosal defects associated with tunneled endoscopy. TTS clips may be combined with a detachable nylon loop or an omental patch for closure of larger defects [7].
- Tunneled exposed EFTR incorporates the following steps: (1) submucosal injection of saline mixed with blue dye 3–5 cm proximal to the tumor; (2) submucosal tunneling to separate the tumor from its covering mucosa; (3) muscle fiber dissection; (4) tumor removal; and (5) tunnel entrance closure (Fig. 4.1) [8].

Non-tunneled Exposed EFTR

- In non-tunneled exposed EFTR, the dissection occurs around a SET with violation of the muscularis propria, followed by defect closure [9]. This method is typically used when the lesion involves the muscularis propria extensively.
- The approach is similar to ESD, using fluid expansion of the submucosal layer to obtain an en bloc resection, and the closure must be full thickness. Multiple techniques have been used for defect closure including loop and clip, OTSC (for defects <2 cm), or endoscopic suturing.

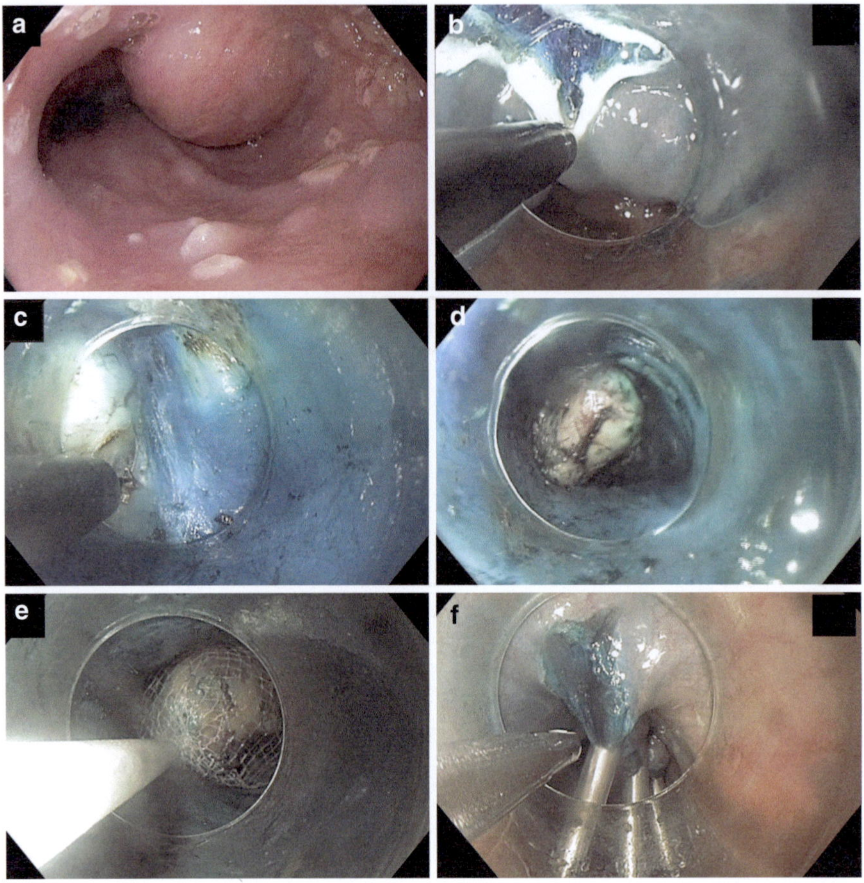

Fig. 4.1 Tunneled exposed EFTR: (**a**) Protruding tumor with a smooth surface. (**b**) Mucosal incision. (**c**) Submucosal tunneling with injection of saline–blue dye mixture. (**d**) Circumferential dissection through muscle fibers around tumor. (**e**) Tumor retrieval. (**f**) Tunnel entrance closure using TTS clips

- Non-tunneled exposed EFTR incorporates the following steps: (1) submucosal injection of normal saline mixed with blue dye for tumor delineation; (2) mucosa incision to access the submucosal plane; (3) submucosal dissection; (4) muscle fiber dissection; (5) tumor removal; and (6) defect closure (seen in Fig. 4.2).

Nonexposed EFTR

- In nonexposed EFTR, the lesion is invaginated into the lumen to allow serosa-to-serosa apposition prior to performing full-thickness resection.

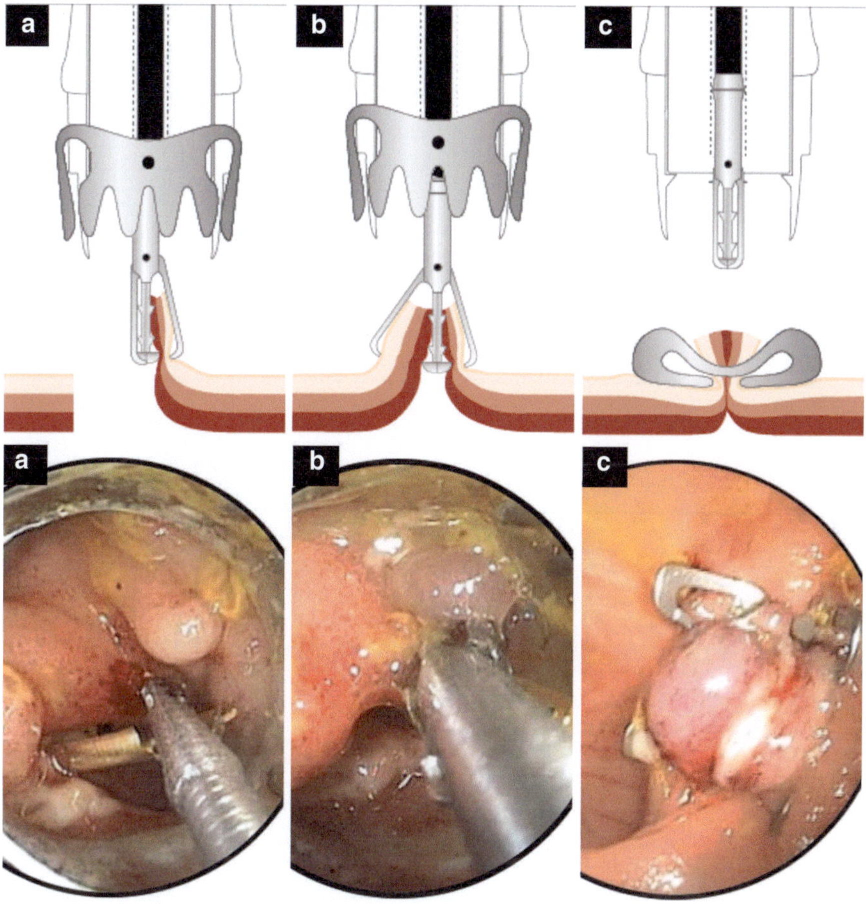

Fig. 4.2 Non-tunneled exposed EFTR closure (schematic via Ovesco, Endoscopy; In Vivo Picture Source: Dr. Thomas Kratt, Interventional Endoscopy, Klinik für Allgemeine, Viszeral- und Transplantationschirurgie, University Hospital Tuebingen, Germany): (**a**) Grasping first perforation edge with first jaw part. (**b**) Grasping second perforation edge with second jaw part, holding both edges simultaneously. (**c**) Clip application with perforation closure

- The full-thickness resection device (FTRD; Ovesco Endoscopy) is the most commonly used all-in-one tool. It has more often been used in the colon due to the diameter of the device; however, reports also show its use for gastric and duodenal lesions [10, 11]. The FTRD contains an applicator cap carrying a modified 14-mm OTSC that can be mounted over a standard colonoscope.
- Nonexposed EFTR incorporates the following steps, outlined in Figs. 4.3 and 4.4: (1) circumferential lesion marking; (2) insertion of FTRD and lesion adjustment; (3) mobilization of lesion and retraction of lesion into device cap; (4) application of OTSC; and (5) resection of tissue and retrieval of specimen.

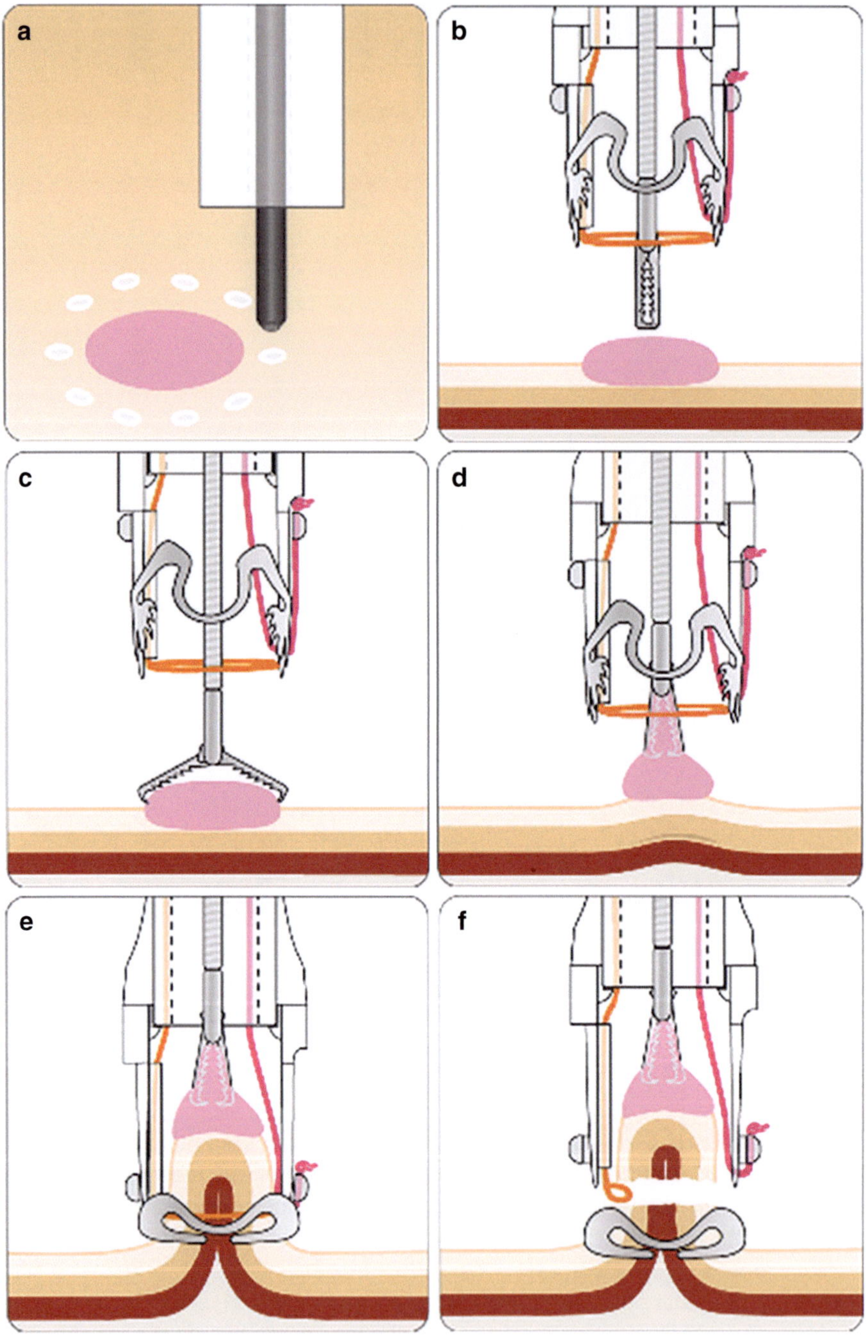

Fig. 4.3 Full-thickness resection device (FTRD) schematic (Ovesco, Endoscopy): (A) Marking of the lesion with a marking probe. (**b**) Insertion of FTRD and adjustment of lesion. (**c**, **d**) Grasping and mobilization of lesion. (**e**) Retraction of lesion into cap with clip application. (**f**) Resection of tissue and retrieval of specimen

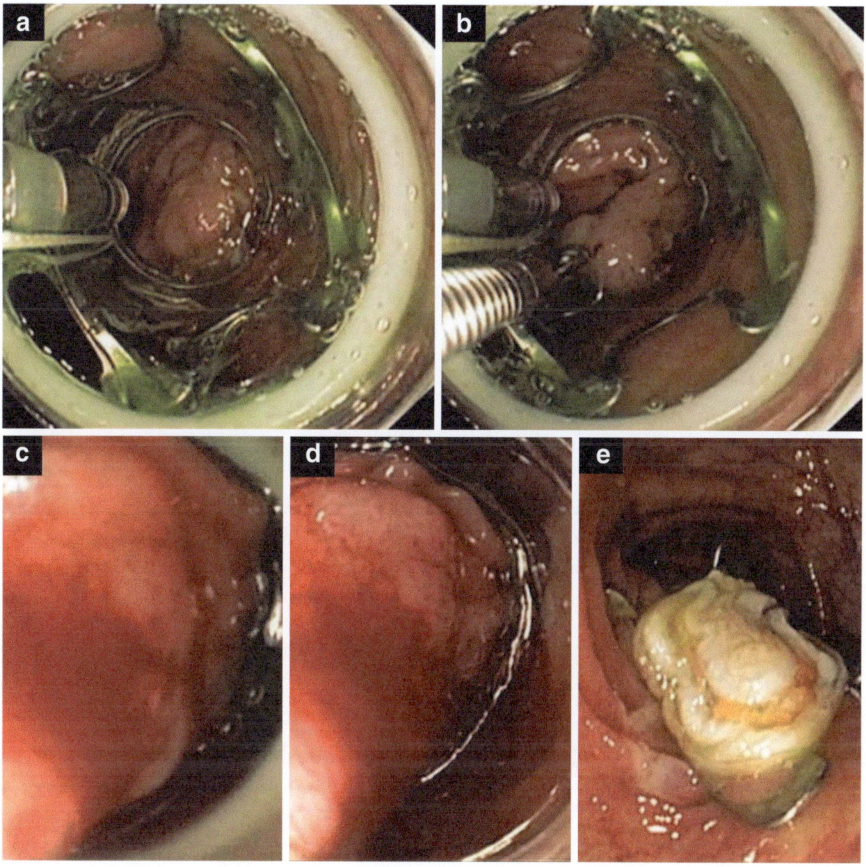

Fig. 4.4 Nonexposed FTRD (Ovesco, Endoscopy): (**a**) Marking of the lesion with a marking probe. (**b**) Grasping and adjustment of lesion. (**c**) Retraction of lesion into device cap. (**d**) Clip application. (**e**) Resection site after tissue removal. (Source: Prof. K. Caca and Dr. A. Schmidt, Klinikum Ludwigsburg, Dept. of Internal Medicine, Gastroenterology, Hemato Onkology, Diabetes and Infektious Diseases, Germany)

Postoperative Care [8, 12]

- After the procedure, patients are typically admitted under observation to monitor for abdominal pain, signs of peritonitis, or hemorrhage, along with diet advancement. Patients are typically kept NPO for 24 h and then placed on clear liquids with gradual diet advancement as tolerated.
- A barium swallow leak test can be used prior to initiating a diet. This depends on the location of resection and is institution-dependent.
- Antibiotics for enteric flora are optional but when used are typically given for 24–48 hours postoperatively.

- Proton pump inhibitors are routinely administered if EFTR was performed in upper GI tract.
- Patients have routine follow-up scheduled to discuss pathology reports and to schedule further management with repeat endoscopy/imaging.

Outcomes

Tunneled Exposed EFTR (i.e., STER)

- A retrospective single-center study of 180 upper GI SETs arising from the muscularis propria demonstrated that en bloc resection was achieved in 90.6% of cases. Median procedure time was 45 min (range 15–200 min). The adverse event rate was 8.3% and included pneumothorax and/or hydrothorax (5.5%), major bleeding (1.1%), and esophageal–pleural fistula (0.6%). There were no treatment-related deaths. Larger tumor size and irregular shape were associated with piecemeal resection and longer procedure duration [13].

Non-tunneled Exposed EFTR

- A prospective, single-center, non-randomized clinical trial containing 68 patients with a total of 66 gastric or colorectal SETs and 2 early-stage colorectal cancers were treated with EFTR. They had an R0 resection rate of 98.5%. Sixty-seven patients required only one OTSC for closure with one patient requiring two OTSC. The adverse event rate was 16.2%, which included abdominal pain (26.5%), local self-resolving peritonitis (2.9%), and bleeding (1.5%). No adverse events required surgical intervention [14].

Nonexposed EFTR

- A prospective multicenter study of 181 colonic lesions treated with a FTRD showed that resection was technically successful in 89.5% of cases, with an R0 resection rate of 76.9%. The R0 resection rate was higher with lesions ≤ 2 cm than in those >2 cm (81.2% vs 58.1%, $P = 0.0038$). The adverse event rate was 9.9%, which included perforation (3.3%) and bleeding (2.2%). Emergency surgery was required in four patients (2.2%) [15].

Comparison Study

- A retrospective single-center study of 46 gastric GISTs treated with exposed non-tunneled EFTR ($n = 32$) or STER ($n = 20$) identified no difference in operative time (94.9 vs 84.9 mins; $P = 0.401$), but the en bloc resection rate for EFTR was significantly higher than for STER (100% vs 80%; $P = 0.029$), while there was no difference in the local recurrence. Additionally, there was no difference in adverse event rate between the two groups; however, patients after STER had earlier resumption of diet and a shorter hospital stay [16].

Pearls	Pitfalls
In efforts to prevent gas complications, which are the most prevalent type of complication encountered in most studies, CO_2 insufflation is imperative (as opposed to air) for any of the EFTR procedures.	Other complications for which to be cognizant depending on location: Abdominal leakage, thoracic effusion, post-operative bleeding, injury to adjacent viscera/vasculature, incomplete resection, and GERD if resection is at the lower esophageal sphincter.
When resecting tumors in the esophagogastric junction, it is easy to lose orientation when establishing your tunnel, so it is important to repeatedly confirm the location of the tumor. Injection of submucosal dye-enhanced saline can help greatly in maintaining orientation.	
It is very difficult to establish a tunnel in the gastric fundus. For SETs in this location, ESD may be a better option.	

References

1. Schurr MO, Buess G, Raestrup H, Arezzo A, Buerkert A, Schell C, et al. Full thickness resection device (FTRD) for endoluminal removal of large bowel tumours: development of the instrument and related experimental studies. Minim Invasive Ther Allied Technol. 2001;10(6):301–9. Available from: https://pubmed.ncbi.nlm.nih.gov/16754033/
2. Kirschniak A, Subotova N, Zieker D, Königsrainer A, Kratt T. The over-the-scope clip (OTSC) for the treatment of gastrointestinal bleeding, perforations, and fistulas. Surg Endosc. 2011;25(9):2901–5. Available from: https://pubmed.ncbi.nlm.nih.gov/21424197/
3. Kiesslich R, Wang TD. Endoscopic full-thickness resection using a novel over-the-scope device. Gastroenterology. 2014;147:740–2. Available from: https://doi.org/10.1053/j.gastro.2014.07.045
4. Andrisani G, Soriani P, Manno M, Pizzicannella M, Pugliese F, Mutignani M, et al. Colo-rectal endoscopic full-thickness resection (EFTR) with the over-the-scope device (FTRD®): a multicenter Italian experience. Dig Liver Dis. 2019;51(3):375–81. Available from: https://pubmed.ncbi.nlm.nih.gov/30377063/

5. Aepli P, Criblez D, Baumeler S, Borovicka J, Frei R. Endoscopic full thickness resection (EFTR) of colorectal neoplasms with the full thickness resection device (FTRD): clinical experience from two tertiary referral centers in Switzerland. United European Gastroenterol J. 2018;6(3):463–70. Available from: https://pubmed.ncbi.nlm.nih.gov/29774161/
6. Ye LP, Zhang Y, Mao XL, Zhu LH, Zhou X, Chen JY. Submucosal tunneling endoscopic resection for small upper gastrointestinal subepithelial tumors originating from the muscularis propria layer. Surg Endosc. 2014;28:524–30.
7. Mönkemüller K, Sarker S, Baig KRKK. Endoscopic creation of an omental patch with an over-the-scope clip system after endoscopic excavation and resection of a large gastrointestinal stromal tumor of the stomach. Endoscopy. 2014;46(Suppl 1):E451–2. Available from: https://pubmed.ncbi.nlm.nih.gov/25314189/
8. Zhang X, Modayil R, Criscitelli T, Stavropoulos SN. Endoscopic resection for subepithelial lesions – pure endoscopic full-thickness resection and submucosal tunneling endoscopic resection. Transl Gastroenterol Hepatol. 2019;4(May):39.
9. Visrodia K, Sethi A. How to learn and perform endoscopic submucosal dissection and full-thickness resection in the colorectum in the United States. Gastrointest Endosc Clin N Am. 2019;29(4):647–57. Available from: https://pubmed.ncbi.nlm.nih.gov/31445688/
10. Meier B, Schmidt A, Glaser N, Meining A, Walter B, Wannhoff A, et al. Endoscopic full-thickness resection of gastric subepithelial tumors with the gFTRD-system: a prospective pilot study (RESET trial). Surg Endosc. 2020;34(2):853–60. Available from: https://pubmed.ncbi.nlm.nih.gov/31187233/
11. Bauder M, Schmidt A, Caca K. Endoscopic full-thickness resection of duodenal lesions-a retrospective analysis of 20 FTRD cases. United European Gastroenterol J. 2018;6(7):1015–21. Available from: https://pubmed.ncbi.nlm.nih.gov/30228889/
12. Ren Z, Lin SL, Zhou PH, Cai SL, Qi ZP, Li J, Yao LQ. Endoscopic full-thickness resection (EFTR) without laparoscopic assistance for nonampullary duodenal subepithelial lesions: our clinical experience of 32 cases. Surg Endosc. 2019;33:3605–11.
13. Chen T, Zhou PH, Chu Y, Zhang YQ, Chen WF, Ji Y, et al. Long-term outcomes of submucosal tunneling endoscopic resection for upper gastrointestinal submucosal tumors. Ann Surg. 2017;265(2):363–9. Available from: https://journals.lww.com/annalsofsurgery/fulltext/2017/02000/long_term_outcomes_of_submucosal_tunneling.20.aspx
14. Guo JT, Zhang JJ, Wu YF, Liao Y, Wang YD, Zhang BZ, et al. Endoscopic full-thickness resection using an over-the-scope device: a prospective study. World J Gastroenterol. 2021;27(8):725.
15. Schmidt A, Beyna T, Schumacher B, Meining A, Richter-Schrag HJ, Messmann H, et al. Colonoscopic full-thickness resection using an over-the-scope device: a prospective multicentre study in various indications. Gut. 2018;67(7):1280–9. Available from: https://pubmed.ncbi.nlm.nih.gov/28798042/
16. Chiu PWY, Yip HC, Chan SM, Ng SKK, Teoh AYB, Ng EKW. Endoscopic full-thickness resection (EFTR) compared to submucosal tunnel endoscopic resection (STER) for treatment of gastric gastrointestinal stromal tumors. Endosc Int Open. 2023;11(2):E179. Available from: /pmc/articles/PMC9949978/

Chapter 5
Peroral Tumorectomy (POET)

Tarik K. Yuce and Kyle A. Perry

Background

- Esophageal submucosal lesions represent a challenging diagnostic and therapeutic dilemma historically requiring repeated surveillance procedures or transthoracic or transgastric surgical resections that carry significant morbidity risk [1].
- Endoscopic resection of submucosal tumors, or peroral tumorectomy (POET), was first described in 2012 for the resection of submucosal tumors originating from the muscularis propria [2]. POET was inspired by previously reported procedures based on endoscopic tunneling techniques, particularly the peroral endoscopic myotomy (POEM).
- This procedure can be safely used to resect challenging submucosal tumors in the esophagus, esophagogastric junction (EGJ), and gastric cardia [3]. POET allows for en bloc resection of tumors arising from the muscularis propria, thereby aiding in establishing the diagnosis of lesions while also potentially achieving curative resection [4]. This technique provides a far less invasive alternative to surgical resection of these lesions.
- Whilc cndoscopic mucosal and full-thickncss rcscctions havc both bccn uscd to treat submucosal tumors, POET provides the advantage of leaving the mucosa directly over the lesion intact [5].

T. K. Yuce · K. A. Perry (✉)
Department of Surgery, Wexner Medical Center, The Ohio State University, Columbus, OH, USA
e-mail: Tarik.Yuce@osumc.edu; Kyle.Perry@osumc.edu

M. Ujiki, Z. M. Callahan (eds.), *Third Space Endoscopy*,
https://doi.org/10.1007/978-3-031-84509-3_5

Indications

- Indications for POET include suspected/confirmed gastrointestinal stromal tumor (GIST) and leiomyoma of the esophagus, EGJ, or gastric cardia [6].
- Particular attention should be paid to lesions that are 2–5 cm in size, causing symptoms, and enlarging on follow-up or have high-risk features noted on biopsy/EUS/CT [7].
- Submucosal lesions less than 2 cm in size may be better suited to surveillance with EUS/endoscopy given their low risk [1].
- Patients who are elderly or have multiple comorbidities which would preclude them from undergoing surgical resection of submucosal lesions of the esophagus/EGJ/cardia may also benefit from the use of POET.
- Suspected or confirmed malignancy is a contraindication for POET [1].

Patient Evaluation

Initial Evaluation

- Absolute contraindications to POET include inability to tolerate general anesthesia due to medical conditions and uncorrectable coagulopathy.

Diagnostic Studies

- Patients should undergo routine preoperative examination using EUS to confirm tumor location, size, and origin within the muscularis propria [8].
- Preoperative contrast-enhanced CT imaging should also be obtained to ensure no evidence of metastatic disease, provide information regarding adjacent anatomic structures such as vessels, and further characterize tumor size and location.

Technique

Procedure Setup and Equipment

- Patients are placed on the operating room table in the supine position and given preoperative antibiotics.
- These procedures should be performed under general anesthesia with endotracheal intubation. Care should be taken to secure the endotracheal tube as far to

the right as possible to allow repeated passage of the endoscope and minimize the risk tube dislodgement.

- The operating endoscopist is positioned to the patient's left side, and an endoscopic assistant stands to the surgeons left to operate the endoscopic instruments utilized during the procedure. If available, a second assistant positioned at the head of the table can stabilize the endoscope during submucosal dissection. POET is performed using a high-definition forward-viewing single-channel endoscope with CO_2 insufflation. A transparent oblique cap is placed on the end of the endoscope to facilitate entry into and dissection of the submucosal tunnel.
- Other equipment that should be available for the procedure include:
  - A generator and hybrid knife system or insulated tip knife.
  - Endoscopic injection needle with indigo carmine injection solution with or without epinephrine.
  - Coagulation grasper.
  - Endoscopic net and large tripod grasper.
  - Endoscopic clips or endoscopic suturing device.

Operative Steps (Fig. 5.1)

- The procedure begins with a diagnostic endoscopy including complete evaluation of the esophagus, EGJ, and cardia in order to confirm location of the submucosal tumor and clear the esophagus and stomach of any fluid or food debris.
- A mucosal lift using injection of 10 mL of indigo carmine solution (0.2 mg/mL) is created approximately 5 cm above the submucosal tumor.
- A 2 cm longitudinal mucosal incision is made at this point, and the endoscope is introduced into the submucosal plane. A tunnel is created in the same fashion to tunnel creation in POEM.
- The submucosal tunnel is carried to and beyond the distal margin of the tumor using serial injection of indigo carmine solution and electrocautery. Once the submucosal tumor is completely visualized and separated from the overlying mucosa, it is dissected free of any adherent muscle fibers and enucleated using electrocautery.
- The tumor can be removed using an endoscopic net or large tripod grasper to withdraw it from the submucosal tunnel and extract transorally.
- Following confirmation of hemostasis, the proximal mucosal entry site is then closed using clips or endoscopic suturing.

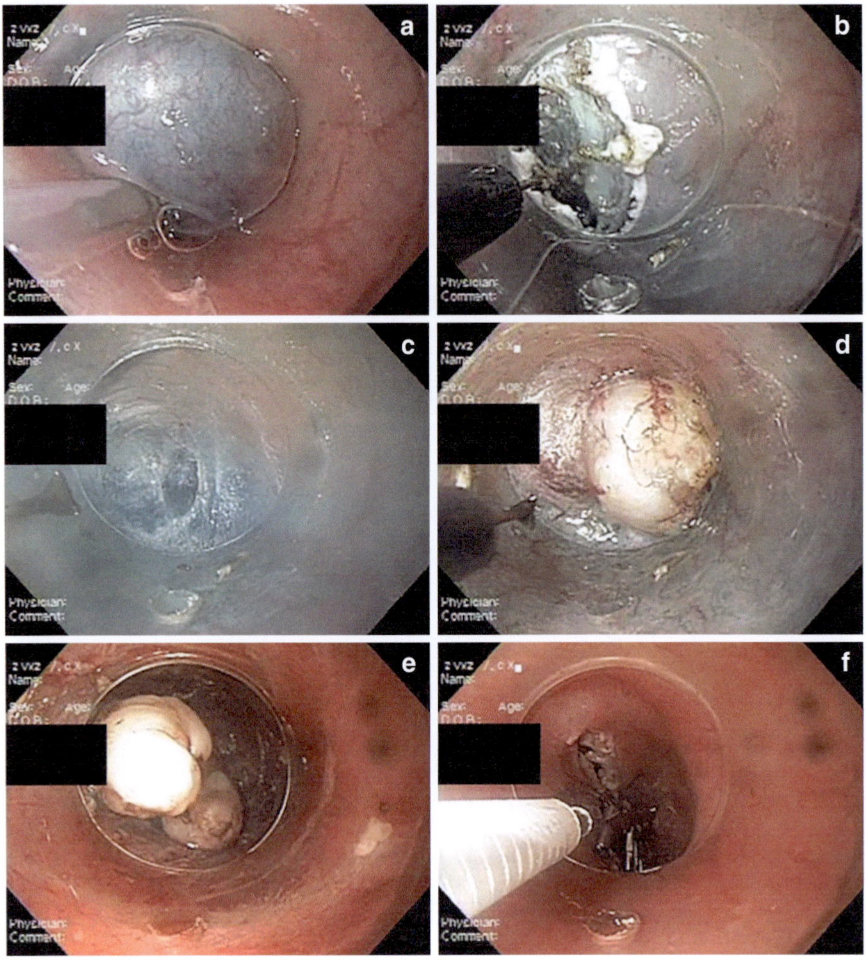

Fig. 5.1 Key steps for peroral tumorectomy. (**a**) Mucosal lift using injection of dilute indigo carmine solution. (**b**) Longitudinal mucosal incision made to gain access to submucosal plane. (**c**) Submucosal tunnel dissected using electrocautery. (**d**) Tumor identified. (**e**) Tumor dissected free of submucosal attachments. (**f**) Proximal mucosal entry site closed using clips

Postoperative Care

- Following the procedure, patients may be admitted and kept NPO overnight. Patients are monitored for any complaints of abdominal or chest pain, dyspnea, abdominal distention, fever, pleural effusion, and subcutaneous emphysema.
- An upper GI contrast study or upper endoscopy may be performed on postoperative day one to evaluate for leak and mucosal integrity. Our practice has been to utilize these selectively in the setting of clinical findings concerning for leak.

- Patients are advanced to clear liquids on postoperative day one then advanced to a full liquid diet for 5 days and are usually discharged from the hospital on postoperative day one or two. Patients begin a soft diet on postoperative day six and return to a regular diet 2 weeks after the procedure.
- Patients should be started on proton pump inhibitors following the procedure and continue for 4 weeks postoperatively.
- When performed for GIST, annual upper endoscopy should be performed for postoperative surveillance, though some have described performing upper endoscopies every 3–6 months for the first year after POET.
- Specimens are sent for histopathologic evaluation, and adjustments to postoperative medications and surveillance may be made based on results.

Outcomes

- Previous reports of postoperative outcomes following POET indicate low rates of complications [9]. Patients who undergo POET may develop postoperative hemorrhage (<1%), subcutaneous emphysema (15–20%), pneumothorax (5–8%), pleural effusion (1–3%), and pneumoperitoneum (1–4%) [10].
- Most patients with subcutaneous emphysema and pneumomediastinum experience resolution with conservative management.
- Pneumothorax and pleural effusions may require temporary closed thoracic drainage depending on patient symptoms (dyspnea, low oxygen saturation).
- En bloc resection rates are reported to be 83–100% [6]. Long-term results show high rates of no residual tumor, no local tumor recurrence, and no distant metastasis.

Pearls	
Anatomy	Care should be taken to identify pertinent anatomic landmarks prior to making the first cut. These include the tumor, EGJ, spine, and aortic arch
Appropriate equipment	Ensuring the appropriate equipment prior to initiation of the procedure is critical. Important tools include the transparent oblique endoscopic cap, appropriate generator with hybrid or insulated tip knife, endoscopic injection needle, coagulation grasper, and endoscopic clips. In cases of difficult esophageal intubation, the use of an overtube may facilitate scope passage and specimen extraction
Tunnel formation	Submucosal tunnel creation should start 5 cm proximal to the lesion. Once in the submucosal plane, attentiveness to the orientation of the circular muscle bundles is critical. Care should be taken to remain within the avascular plane until the tumor is visualized. Complete dissection of the mucosal side of the lesion prior to division of muscular wall attachments reduces the risk of mucosal injury at the level of the tumor

(continued)

Specimen extraction	These tumors can typically be extracted using a large endoscopic tripod grasper. In the case of larger lesions, it may be more secure to utilize an endoscopic net to secure the tumor prior to removal. In these cases, an endoscopic grasper can facilitate removal from the submucosal tunnel and a net can be used to secure it within the esophageal or gastric lumen prior to final extraction
Pitfalls	
Cap fixation	The oblique endoscopic resection cap should be secured in place using instrument tape to prevent cap dislodgement during dissection of the submucosal space
Insufflation	CO_2 insufflation should be used for all submucosal tunneling procedures including POET. Use of air for insufflation carries an increased risk of symptomatic pneumothorax requiring tube thoracostomy. Pneumoperitoneum is common during the performance of these procedures, and the abdominal examination should be monitored during the procedure, particularly because most endoscopic insufflation systems do not monitor pressure. Clinically apparent pneumoperitoneum should be managed with needle decompression
Submucosal tunnel bleeding	Bleeding within the submucosal tunnel may hamper visualization and increase risk of inadvertently injuring surrounding structures. Should bleeding occur, use of pulse irrigation with gentle suctioning may allow for the visualization of the source. Tamponading the vessel using the endoscope or transparent cap may also allow for identification of the source. Precise coagulation using coagulation forceps can then be used. Severe bleeding may require placement of a Blakemore-Sengstaken tube
Full thickness injury	Unintended mucosotomy at the level of the tumor may result in a full thickness esophageal perforation. In this case, careful attention must be paid to complete mucosal closure. With small mucosal injuries, this can be achieved with standard endoscopic clips. However, in the case of larger defects, consideration should be given to closure with endoscopic suturing or an over-the-scope clip device. Postoperative esophagram should be obtained on postoperative day zero or one to ensure secure mucosal closure

References

1. Eleftheriadis N. Submucosal tunnel endoscopy: Peroral endoscopic myotomy and peroral endoscopic tumor resection. World J Gastrointest Endosc. 2016;8(2):86.
2. Gong W, Xiong Y, Zhi F, Liu S, Wang A, Jiang B. Preliminary experience of endoscopic submucosal tunnel dissection for upper gastrointestinal submucosal tumors. Endoscopy. 2012;44(3):231–5.
3. Onimaru M, Inoue H, Bechara R, Tanabe M, Abad MRA, Ueno A, et al. Clinical outcomes of per-oral endoscopic tumor resection for submucosal tumors in the esophagus and gastric cardia. Dig Endosc. 2020;32(3):328–36.
4. Liu BR, Song JT, Kong LJ, Pei FH, Wang XH, Du YJ. Tunneling endoscopic muscularis dissection for subepithelial tumors originating from the muscularis propria of the esophagus and gastric cardia. Surg Endosc. 2013;27(11):4354–9.
5. Inoue H, Ikeda H, Hosoya T, Onimaru M, Yoshida A, Eleftheriadis N, et al. Submucosal endoscopic tumor resection for subepithelial tumors in the esophagus and cardia. Endoscopy. 2012;44(3):225–30.

6. Liu BR, Song JT. Submucosal tunneling endoscopic resection (STER) and other novel applications of submucosal tunneling in humans. Gastrointest Endosc Clin N Am. 2016;26(2):271–82.
7. Chung CS, Chen KH, Chen KC, Chen CY, Lee TH, Lin CK, et al. Peroral endoscopic tumor resection (POET) with preserved mucosa technique for management of upper gastrointestinal tract subepithelial tumors. Surg Endosc. 2021;35(7):3753–62.
8. Chiu PWY, Yip HC, Teoh AYB, Wong VWY, Chan SM, Wong SKH, et al. Per oral endoscopic tumor (POET) resection for treatment of upper gastrointestinal subepithelial tumors. Surg Endosc. 2019;33(4):1326–33.
9. Du C, Chai NL, Ling-Hu EQ, Li ZJ, Li LS, et al. Submucosal tunneling endoscopic resection: an effective and safe therapy for upper gastrointestinal submucosal tumors originating from the muscularis propria layer. World J Gastroenterol. 2019;25(2):245–57.
10. Wang XY, Xu MD, Yao LQ, Zhou PH, Pleskow D, Li QL, et al. Submucosal tunneling endoscopic resection for submucosal tumors of the esophagogastric junction originating from the muscularis propria layer: a feasibility study (with videos). Surg Endosc. 2014;28(6):1971–7.

Part II
Intentional Scar Formation

Chapter 6
Anti-reflux Mucosectomy (ARMS)

Mason Hedberg and Derrius Anderson

Background

- The anti-reflux mucosectomy (ARMS) procedure was discovered in 2003 when a patient with Barrett's esophagus at the gastroesophageal junction (GEJ) underwent an endoscopic mucosal resection and had improvement of their symptoms [1]. In 2014, the same team published a case series of ten patients who underwent an ARMS procedure with improvement of their gastroesophageal reflux disease (GERD) symptoms and DeMeester scores [2].
- Since then, it has been shown in quality-of-life metrics and objective reflux data that ARMS can serve as a promising tool for anti-reflux interventions. ARMS is also a useful procedure for patients with a history of sleeve gastrectomy with refractory GERD who are unable to or refuse conversion to RYGB [3, 4]. ARMS is useful for patients who have previously undergone surgical intervention for GERD and TIF [5].

Indications

- ARMS is indicated in patients who have failed medical management of GERD electing for anti-reflux procedure or patients who are unable to tolerate PPIs due to medication interactions or side effects.

M. Hedberg (✉)
Department of Surgery, Endeavor Health, Evanston, IL, USA
e-mail: hhedberg@northshore.org

D. Anderson
University of Chicago Medicine, Chicago, IL, USA

M. Ujiki, Z. M. Callahan (eds.), *Third Space Endoscopy*,
https://doi.org/10.1007/978-3-031-84509-3_6

- Contraindications include a significant hiatal hernia (>2 cm) and abnormal peristalsis on high-resolution manometry.

Patient Evaluation

Initial Evaluation

- A thorough history and physical should be performed with a particular emphasis on duration and severity of symptoms.
- Prior endoscopic reports should be reviewed, noting prior strictures, evidence of esophagitis, or Barrett's esophagus.

Diagnostic Studies

- Patient evaluation includes objective testing of the esophagus and stomach. Patients should undergo barium esophagram to assess for hiatal hernia as well as upper endoscopy to confirm the absence of anatomical abnormalities or pathologies of the stomach and esophagus. GERD is diagnosed with a pH probe study to quantify the degree of acid reflux; this can be excluded in the presence of severe (Los Angeles grade C or D) esophagitis. Lastly, esophageal manometry is performed to rule out a primary esophageal motility disorder.
- Patients with medically refractory GERD or those who desired the ability to discontinue PPIs were considered candidates to undergo ARMS.

Preoperative Preparation

- We perform ARMS in the operating room under general anesthesia. In this setting, while highly unlikely, rapid conversion to laparoscopic or open surgery is possible in the event of gastric perforation or bleeding that cannot be controlled endoscopically.
- The patient is given mechanical venous thromboembolism prophylaxis only.

Technique

Endoscopic Access and Anatomical Landmarks

- The patient is positioned supine with arms at the side. The endotracheal tube should emanate from the patient's right with the operator at the patient's left. An endoscopic bite block should be in place to protect the lips from injury between the teeth and endoscope.
- Careful inspection of the gastroesophageal junction should be performed in ante and retroflexion to confirm the absence of significant hiatal hernia (<2 cm longitudinally or > Hill grade II) and other pathology such as ulceration or masses.
- We routinely perform endoluminal planimetry at the start of the case to establish a baseline for future post-procedure comparison.

Endoscopic Planning

- After initial assessments, the scope is removed and is fitted with the banded endoscopic mucosal resection (EMR) system (Fig. 6.1). Typically, six bands are included on a cap, and the intent is to fire three bands each on the anterior and posterior gastric cardia, resecting the mucosa and leaving bridges of intact mucosa at the greater and lesser curves (Fig. 6.2). The spared mucosa on the lesser curve helps avoid dysphagia requiring endoscopic dilation.
- The EMR snare with electrocautery can be used to mark the extent of the anterior and posterior resections, which provides guidance when anatomy and visualization becomes distorted as the procedure progresses (Fig. 6.3).

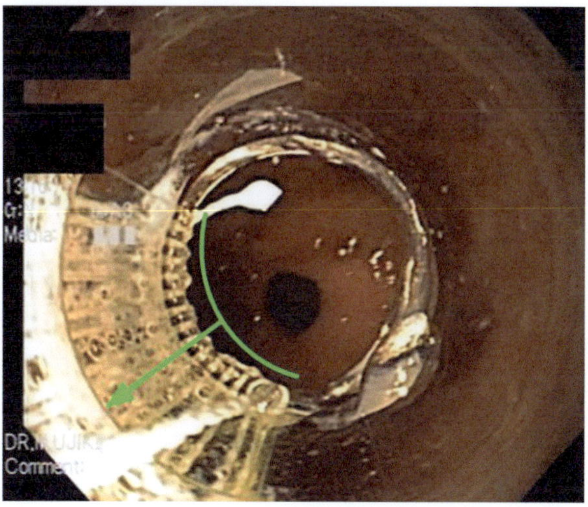

Fig. 6.1 Banded EMR cap in place. The bands are centered on the accessory channel for the most direct path to the deploying mechanism

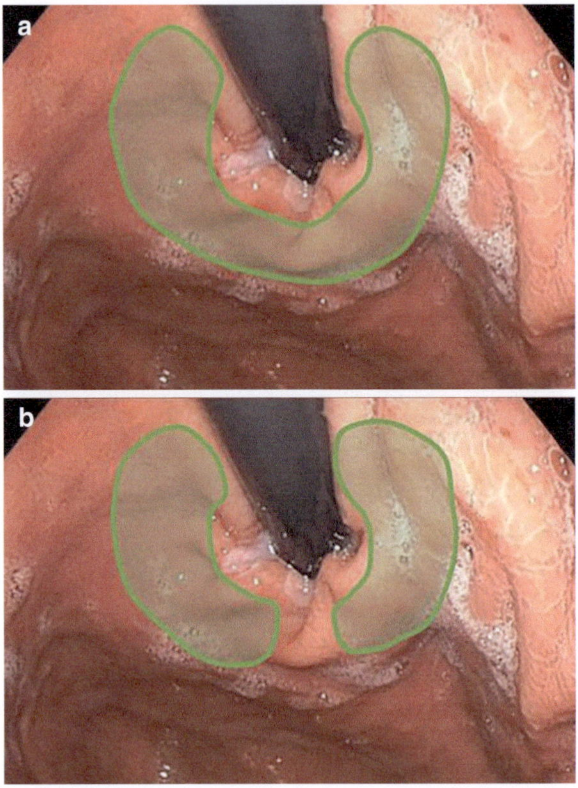

Fig. 6.2 Scope in retroflexion, areas of resection marked out. (**a**) Original procedure as described, sparing only greater curvature. (**b**) Modified technique to decrease the rate of postoperative dysphagia requiring dilation. (Used with permission from Wong et al. [8])

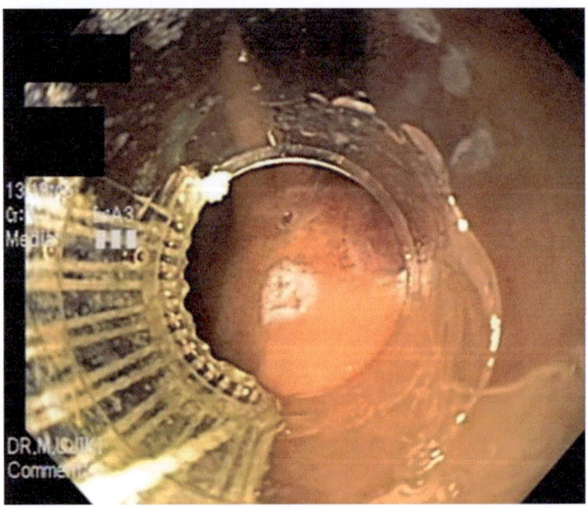

Fig. 6.3 Anterior area of resection marked with electrocautery

- We use a mixture of saline and indigo carmine as a mucosal lift agent (1 mL in 500 mL saline). A single resection begins with injection, being aware that the area of resection will extend up to a centimeter circumferentially around the injection site.

Endoscopic Mucosal Resection

- We begin resection on the anterior surface of the stomach 2 cm from the lesser curve and proceed in a counterclockwise fashion around the GEJ, sparing a bridge at the greater curve.
- Achieving mucosal lift requires the needle tip be within the submucosal space. Sometimes the needle must be advanced or retracted slightly after injection begins to access the correct space. Once lift begins, continue to inject another 2–3 cc only (Fig. 6.4). Too much solution can limit the amount of mucosa that is captured by the band.
- After injection, the needle is removed (to maximize suction capability), and the cap is pressed onto the mucosa to suction the lifted bubble into the cap. The mucosa will thin and the blue dye will be visible. If the lift was executed well, the mucosa should fill the entire cap and come all the way to the lens of the scope (Fig. 6.5). Once adequate mucosa is captured, a band is deployed. If an adequate amount of mucosa was captured, the mucosa will be pinched in under the band (Fig. 6.6).
- The snare is passed through the scope and the banded mucosa is snared. Ideally, the snare is placed below the band, which will result in the largest resection possible (Fig. 6.7). Snaring above the band will miss mucosa within the band, and

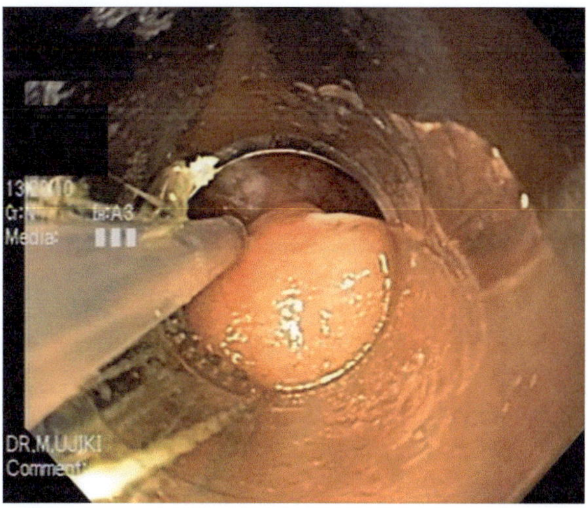

Fig. 6.4 Submucosal lift, 2 3 cc injected once lift begins

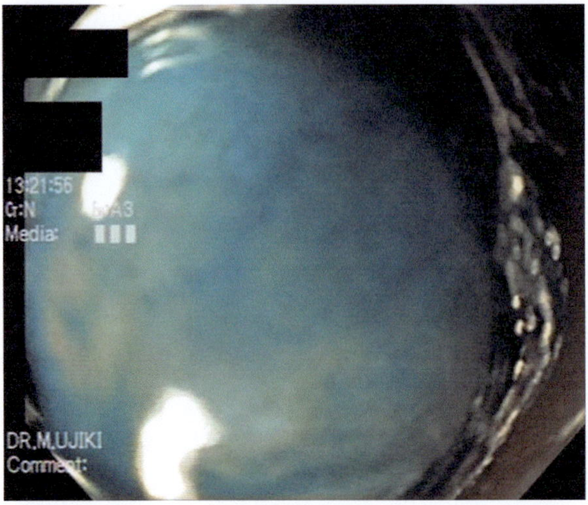

Fig. 6.5 Mucosal "bubble" suctioned into the EMR cap—the blue lifting agent is visible through the thinned mucosa

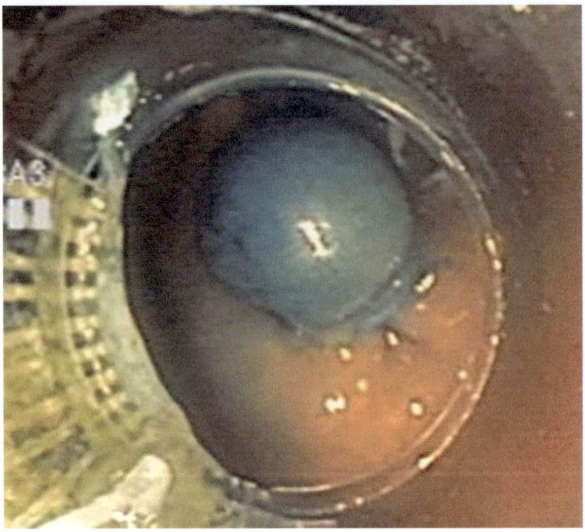

Fig. 6.6 Band deployed—the mucosa pinched around the base of the band indicates a broad capture

snaring across the band should be avoided to prevent the band from getting stuck on the snare.

- Once the resection is complete, the cap is used to spread the edges of the mucosa to examine the complete area of resection while simultaneously carefully inspecting the submucosa for deeper injuries, visible vessels, and bleeding. Visible vessels are coagulated to prevent a delayed bleed. Figure 6.8 shows the resected area before and after using the cap to spread and inspect.
- The process is repeated to achieve adequate resection of the anterior and posterior gastric cardia (Fig. 6.9). The resected specimens/bands typically collect in the gastric fundus, which can be retrieved with a Roth net.

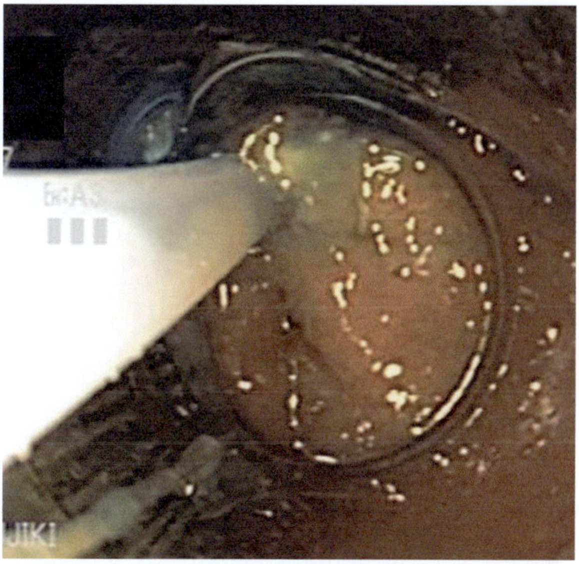

Fig. 6.7 The banded area ensnared below the band to maximize area of resection

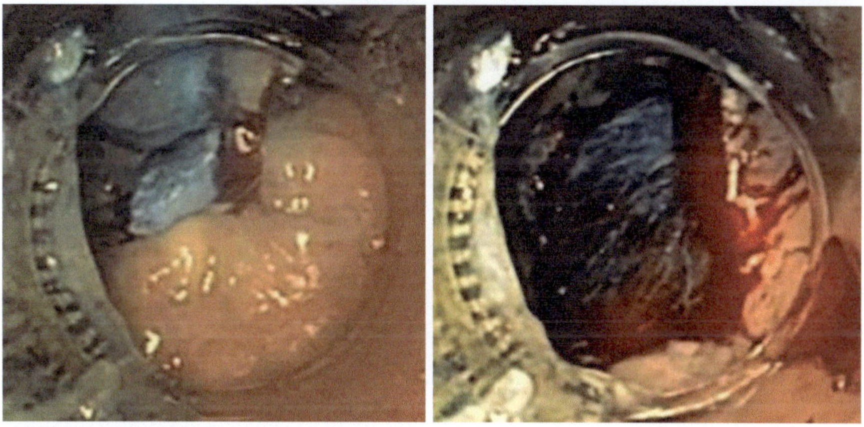

Fig. 6.8 Same area of resection before and after spreading the mucosal edges/inspecting the submucosa with the cap

Postoperative Care

- In recovery, patients are given a clear liquid diet to ensure they can tolerate and swallow appropriately for adequate hydration prior to discharge home. Postoperative diet requires a soft pureed diet for 2 weeks post procedure.
- Proton pump inhibitors can be discontinued the day of surgery or weaned over a few weeks in the postoperative period.

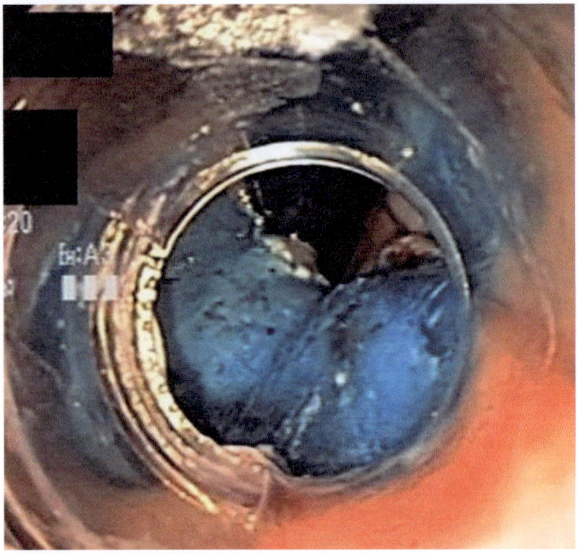

Fig. 6.9 Appearance of multiple contiguous resections

- Pain is typically well controlled with Tylenol and NSAIDs. A weak narcotic can be prescribed for discomfort not well controlled with over-the-counter medications.
- Early dysphagia is typically managed with dietary and lifestyle modifications which will include full liquid or soft diet, chewing food well, and drinking plenty of water with meals. Persistent dysphagia is amenable to balloon dilation.

Outcomes

- Anti-reflux mucosectomy is a technically successful procedure, with success rates of approximately 97% [6, 7].
- Expected clinical response rates measured by discontinuation or decreased use of PPIs are approximately 70% [6, 7].
- Most common complications include dysphagia and bleeding, which occur approximately 11% and 5% of the time, respectively [6, 7].
- The technical feasibility of completing this procedure in patients with previous sleeve gastrectomy is possible with >50% improvement of GERD-HQRL scores [3].
- In patients who have undergone TIF or Nissen fundoplication, this procedure is also feasible with non-standardized documented improvement in symptoms [5].

Pearls	Pitfalls
Check that the endoscope is able to fully retroflex before starting the procedure	Inadequate retroflexion will prevent carrying mucosal resection close to the GEJ
Once a good lift is initiated, inject only ~2 cc. Too much lift can inhibit broad mucosal capture	Too little lift will increase the chances of a muscular/full thickness injury
Sparing a mucosal "bridge" at the lesser and greater curve decreases the risk of dysphagia	Mucosal resection crossing the Z line onto esophageal tissue increases the risk of dysphagia
Positioning the snare completely under the band will maximize the area of mucosal resection	Crossing the band with the snare may require prolonged hot snare application and may divide the band—partial band pieces can get stuck in the suction channel of the scope

References

1. Satodate H, Inoue H, Yoshida T, Usui S, Iwashita M, Fukami N, et al. Circumferential EMR of carcinoma arising in Barrett's esophagus: case report. Gastrointest Endosc. 2003;58(2):288–92. Available from: https://pubmed.ncbi.nlm.nih.gov/12872107/
2. Inoue H, Ito H, Ikeda H, Sato C, Sato H, Phalanusitthepha C, Hayee BH, Eleftheriadis N, Kudo SE. Anti-reflux mucosectomy for gastroesophageal reflux disease in the absence of hiatus hernia: a pilot study. Ann Gastroenterol. 2014;27(4):346.
3. Debourdeau A, Vitton V, Monino L, Barthet M, Gonzalez JM. Antireflux mucosectomy band (ARM-b) in treatment of refractory gastroesophageal reflux disease after bariatric surgery. Obes Surg. 2020;30(11):4654–8. Available from: https://pubmed.ncbi.nlm.nih.gov/32676843/
4. Patil G, Iyer A, Dalal A, Maydeo A. Antireflux mucosectomy for managing reflux symptoms in an obese patient post laparoscopic sleeve gastrectomy. Scand J Gastroenterol. 2019;54(12):1494–7. Available from: https://pubmed.ncbi.nlm.nih.gov/31791169/
5. Randhawa N, Khalyfa A, Khan M, Roebuck C, Inam M, Ayub K. Utilization of antireflux mucosectomy and resection and plication: a novel approach for the management of recurrent gastroesophageal reflux disease after prior nissen fundoplication or transoral incisionless fundoplication. J Clin Med. 2022;11(23):7141.
6. Garg R, Mohammed A, Singh A, Schleicher M, Thota PN, Rustagi T, et al. Anti-reflux mucosectomy for refractory gastroesophageal reflux disease: a systematic review and meta-analysis. Endosc Int Open. 2022;10(6):E854–64. Available from: https://pubmed.ncbi.nlm.nih.gov/35692929/
7. Yeh JH, Lee CT, Hsu MH, Lin CW, Hsiao PJ, Chen CL, et al. Antireflux mucosal intervention (ARMI) procedures for refractory gastroesophageal reflux disease: a systematic review and meta-analysis. Ther Adv Gastroenterol. 2022;15. Available from: https://pubmed.ncbi.nlm.nih.gov/35509424/
8. Wong HJ, Su B, Attaar M, Kuchta K, Stearns S, Linn JG, et al. Anti-reflux mucosectomy (ARMS) results in improved recovery and similar reflux quality of life outcomes compared to laparoscopic Nissen fundoplication. Surg Endosc. 2021;35(12):7174–82. Available from: https://pubmed.ncbi.nlm.nih.gov/33237465/

Chapter 7
Anti-reflux Mucosal Ablation (ARMA)

Mayo Tanabe and Haruhiro Inoue

Background

Gastroesophageal reflux disease (GERD) is one of the most prevalent and challenging gastrointestinal disorders, with its incidence steadily increasing worldwide [1, 2]. Patients with GERD often experience diminished health-related quality of life due to persistent symptoms such as heartburn, regurgitation, and chest discomfort. While proton pump inhibitors (PPIs) remain the cornerstone of GERD treatment, up to 30–40% of patients report persistent symptoms despite optimal medical therapy [3]. This subset of patients, known as PPI-refractory GERD, poses significant clinical and economic challenges, emphasizing the need for alternative therapeutic approaches.

Prolonged dependence on acid suppressive medications has also raised concerns regarding potential side effects, including osteoporosis, hypomagnesemia, and vitamin B12 deficiency [4]. These risks, coupled with the high cost of long-term pharmacotherapy, have spurred interest in minimally invasive interventions that bridge the gap between medical management and surgical options.

Several endoscopic techniques, including transoral incisionless fundoplication, non-ablative radiofrequency treatments, and plication methods, have emerged as viable alternatives for GERD management [5–7]. Among these, anti-reflux mucosectomy (ARMS) [8, 9] and its evolution into anti-reflux mucosal ablation (ARMA) [10, 11] have garnered attention due to their efficacy, simplicity, and safety. ARMS

This chapter is dedicated to all researchers and clinicians advancing the field of minimally invasive GERD therapies.

M. Tanabe (✉) · H. Inoue
Digestive Diseases Center, Showa University Koto Toyosu Hosptital, Tokyo, Japan
e-mail: haru.inoue@med.showa-u.ac.jp

M. Ujiki, Z. M. Callahan (eds.), *Third Space Endoscopy*,
https://doi.org/10.1007/978-3-031-84509-3_7

involves the resection of the gastric cardia mucosa to induce scar formation and enhance the gastroesophageal junction (GEJ) flap valve. Initial studies demonstrated favorable outcomes, with significant symptom relief and improved acid reflux parameters. Building upon the foundational success of ARMS, ARMA utilizes mucosal ablation rather than resection to achieve similar outcomes. This modification simplifies the procedure, reduces the risk of complications such as perforation, and allows for retreatment in cases of prior intervention failure. Preliminary studies on ARMA have shown promising results, with clinical success rates ranging from 58% to 89% and minimal adverse events.

This chapter aims to provide an in-depth exploration of ARMA, including its technical approach, clinical outcomes, and future prospects as a minimally invasive solution for GERD patients who are refractory to medical therapy or seek alternatives to surgery.

Techniques

Anti-reflux mucosal ablation (ARMA) is a minimally invasive endoscopic procedure designed to enhance the function of the gastroesophageal junction (GEJ) by inducing controlled scarring through mucosal ablation. This scarring reshapes the mucosal flap valve, effectively reducing reflux by narrowing the gastric cardia opening. The procedure evolved from anti-reflux mucosectomy (ARMS), retaining its clinical benefits while simplifying the technique to make it safer and more accessible.

Key Features of ARMA

One of the key advantages of ARMA lies in its minimally invasive nature. The procedure is performed using standard endoscopic equipment, and depending on patient needs and physician preference, it can be conducted under general anesthesia with endotracheal intubation or using propofol sedation. This flexibility ensures patient comfort while maintaining procedural safety.

The ablation in ARMA is highly targeted, focusing on the gastric side of the GEJ. Ablation patterns are applied circumferentially or in specific configurations such as a "butterfly" or "horseshoe" shape. These patterns are designed to spare critical areas, minimizing risks like stenosis while effectively reshaping the gastroesophageal flap valve.

ARMA also stands out for its repeatability. Unlike ARMS, which involves mucosal resection and may limit subsequent interventions, ARMA can be safely repeated in cases of prior treatment failure or symptom recurrence. This repeatability provides a significant advantage for managing refractory cases or complications that arise post-treatment.

Lastly, ARMA incorporates advanced safety measures to minimize complications. The use of argon plasma coagulation (APC) or a triangle-tip knife ensures precise ablation while reducing the risk of adverse events, such as perforation. These features make ARMA not only an effective therapeutic option but also a safer alternative for GERD patients requiring endoscopic intervention.

Procedural Steps (Fig. 7.1)

The ARMA procedure begins with retroflexed visualization of the GEJ using a gastroscope equipped with a transparent hood for optimal visibility. Continuous insufflation with CO_2 ensures clear visualization. Ablation is performed using either a triangle-tip knife (spray coagulation 50 W, effect 2) or APC (forced mode, flow 1.0 L/min, 70–100 W). The "butterfly" configuration spares two contralateral areas

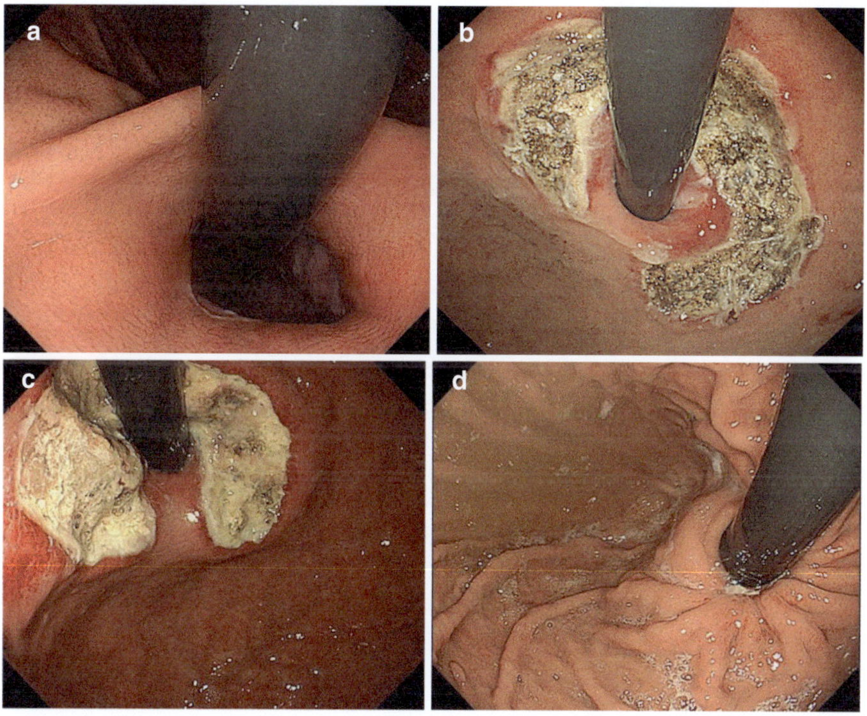

Fig. 7.1 Endoscopic follow-up of anti-reflux mucosal ablation (ARMA). (**a**) Pre-ARMA. Endoscopy in retroflexion demonstrated significant hernia but no sliding component. (**b**) Immediately post-ARMA. Endoscopy in retroflexion showed artificial ulcer in "horseshoe shape." (1 Scope diameter wide normal mucosa left at the greater curvature.) (**c**) Appearance at 4 days post-ARMA. (**d**) Appearance 1 month post-ARMA. Mucosal flap valve was reshaped

of normal mucosa, each approximately one scope diameter in width, to reduce the risk of stenosis.

Post-procedure Care

After ARMA, patients are fasted for 24 h, transitioning to clear fluids and subsequently a regular diet as tolerated. Post-procedural management includes a daily dose of PPIs or potassium-competitive acid blockers (PCABs) for 1 month to support healing and reduce acid exposure during the recovery phase. Patients typically recover well, with follow-up endoscopies performed to monitor healing and assess the effectiveness of the intervention.

Outcomes

Bi-institutional Study Results

Between May 2018 and December 2022, a bi-institutional study evaluated the clinical outcomes and safety of ARMA in patients with GERD who were refractory to acid suppression medications or dependent on such therapies [11]. This retrospective analysis, using prospectively collected data from two international centers, enrolled 68 patients. Of these, definitive GERD was diagnosed in 44 patients (64.7%), while 24 patients (35.3%) exhibited reflux hypersensitivity.

Clinical success, defined as a > 50% reduction in a validated GERD questionnaire, was observed in 60% of patients (39/65) at 2–6 months and in 70% of patients (21/30) at 1 year post-ARMA. The median GERD-HRQL score improved significantly from 26 at baseline to 11 at 2–6 months post-procedure ($p < 0.001$). Among the 51 patients (71.8%) who underwent 24-hour pH monitoring, the median acid exposure time (AET) decreased markedly from 5.3% to 0.7% ($p = 0.003$), with a significant reduction in esophagitis rates ($p < 0.001$).

The study demonstrated ARMA's technical feasibility and reproducibility. Transient stenosis requiring balloon dilation was observed in 13.2% (9 patients), but no severe complications were reported. These findings establish ARMA as a safe and effective treatment option for both reflux hypersensitivity and confirmed GERD patients, regardless of their response to acid suppression therapies.

Meta-analyses

Two comprehensive meta-analyses have recently assessed the efficacy and safety of anti-reflux mucosal interventions (ARMI), including anti-reflux mucosectomy (ARMS), anti-reflux mucosal ablation (ARMA), and anti-reflux band ligation (ARBL), in the treatment of gastroesophageal reflux disease (GERD) [12, 13]. These meta-analyses provide robust evidence supporting ARMI as an effective therapeutic approach for GERD, particularly in patients with refractory symptoms or dependency on proton pump inhibitors (PPIs). The pooled clinical success rate for ARMI procedures across studies was 73.8%, with ARMA demonstrating the highest success rate at 86.7%, outperforming ARMS (68.6%) and ARBL (76.5%). Clinical success was defined as a significant improvement in GERD-related symptoms, quantified through validated GERD-specific questionnaires. These findings highlight the superior efficacy of ARMA compared to other ARMI techniques in achieving meaningful symptom relief. In addition to symptom improvement, ARMA also demonstrated substantial enhancements in GERD-related quality of life. Patients undergoing ARMA reported significant reductions in validated scales such as the GERD-HRQL (Health-Related Quality of Life) and FSSG (Frequency Scale for the Symptoms of GERD), with improvements sustained up to 1 year post-procedure. Objective measures of GERD severity also showed notable improvements. Specifically, ARMA reduced the median acid exposure time (AET) from 5.3% pre-procedure to 0.7% post-procedure and decreased DeMeester scores from 23.0 to 4.2, underscoring its efficacy in acid reflux control. Importantly, ARMA proved effective in reducing long-term PPI dependency. Approximately 64% of patients discontinued PPI therapy within 1 year of undergoing the procedure, addressing both the financial burden and potential adverse effects associated with prolonged PPI use. This reduction in medication reliance represents a significant advantage for patients seeking non-pharmacological solutions to GERD. These meta-analytic findings establish ARMA as a safe, effective, and minimally invasive intervention for GERD. By offering superior clinical success rates, sustained symptom relief, and reduced medication dependency, ARMA occupies a pivotal role in the management of GERD, particularly for patients who are refractory to medical therapy or seek alternatives to invasive surgical procedures. Further randomized controlled trials are warranted to validate these results and refine patient selection criteria.

Positioning ARMA in GERD Management

ARMA represents a highly effective and minimally invasive option for managing GERD in select patient populations. It is particularly suitable for individuals with PPI-refractory GERD who continue to experience symptoms despite optimal pharmacological management. Additionally, ARMA offers an alternative for patients reluctant to undergo invasive surgical procedures, such as Nissen fundoplication, by providing a less invasive approach with comparable symptom relief and acid reduction. Furthermore, ARMA is an ideal option for reducing long-term dependency on PPIs, addressing both the side effects associated with prolonged medication use and the economic burden of chronic therapy. As the most straightforward endoscopic approach, ARMA also allows for retreatment in patients with prior procedural scarring or refractory outcomes, further extending its utility. By effectively balancing efficacy, safety, and feasibility, ARMA occupies a critical niche in the continuum of GERD management.

Future Perspectives(Table 7.1, Fig. 7.2)

As research on ARMA continues to advance, several areas of focus aim to refine and expand its applications. A critical priority is evaluating the long-term outcomes of ARMA to determine the durability of symptom relief and acid control over extended follow-up periods. Another area of interest lies in improving patient selection criteria to identify individuals who are most likely to benefit from ARMA, including those with atypical or refractory GERD symptoms. Additionally, the potential for combining ARMA with other endoscopic or medical treatments presents a promising avenue to enhance therapeutic outcomes. Collaborative studies and larger randomized controlled trials will play a pivotal role in solidifying ARMA's position as a mainstream treatment option for GERD, ensuring that its full potential is realized across diverse patient populations.

Furthermore, advanced techniques such as anti-reflux mucosal plasty (ARM-P) [14] and anti-reflux mucosal plasty with valve (ARM-P/V) [15] are being explored as potential solutions to address post-ARMA challenges, including insufficient therapeutic effects or post-procedural bleeding. These innovative approaches involve closing ulcers immediately during the procedure to optimize outcomes and mitigate risks, potentially expanding the scope and efficacy of ARMA-based interventions. However, ARMA continues to hold a critical position in GERD treatment due to its

Table 7.1 Technical Description of ARMI Procedures

Procedure	Description
Anti-reflux mucosectomy (ARMS)	Mucosal resection at the gastric cardia
Anti-reflux mucosal ablation (ARMA)	Mucosal ablation at the gastric cardia
Anti-reflux band ligation (ARBL)	Rubber bands are employed at the GEJ without resection to achieve tissue ischemia and subsequent mucosal sloughing
Anti-reflux mucoplasty (ARM-P)	Mucosal resection at the gastric cardia + mucosal reconstruction by closure
Anti-reflux mucoplasty with valve (ARM-P/V)	Mucosal resection at the gastric cardia + valve formation using residual mucosa + mucosal reconstruction by closure

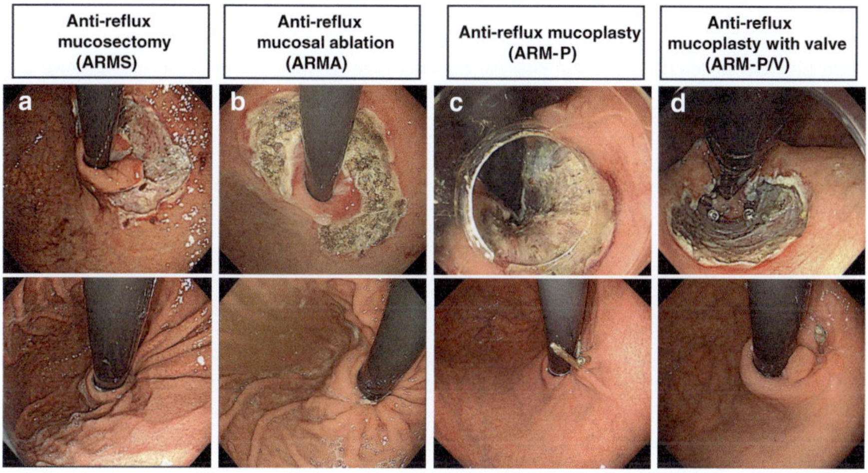

Fig. 7.2 Anti-reflux mucosal intervention (ARMI). (**a**) This figure illustrates four types of anti-reflux mucosal interventions (ARMI): Anti-reflux mucosectomy (ARMS): Mucosal resection at the gastric cardia (top) with post-procedural remodeling of the gastroesophageal junction (bottom). (**b**) Anti-reflux mucosal ablation (ARMA): Thermal ablation at the gastric cardia (top) with post-procedural scar formation enhancing the gastroesophageal flap valve (bottom). (**c**) Anti-reflux mucoplasty (ARM-P): Mucosal resection followed by closure at the gastric cardia (top), resulting in mucosal reconstruction (bottom). (**d**) Anti-reflux mucoplasty with valve (ARM-PV): Mucosal resection with valve formation using residual mucosa and closure (top), leading to enhanced valve function (bottom)

straightforward, minimally invasive approach, which allows for shorter procedure times and excellent repeatability. Its simplicity and adaptability make ARMA an accessible option for a wide range of patients, including those with prior procedural scarring, such as those resulting from previous anti-reflux interventions like ARMS, or refractory outcomes, such as persistent GERD symptoms despite repeated pharmacological or surgical treatments. By addressing GERD effectively with minimal complications, ARMA remains an integral and practical solution within the spectrum of endoscopic therapies.

Conclusion

ARMA represents a significant advancement in GERD treatment, providing a safe, effective, and minimally invasive option for patients with refractory symptoms. Its simplicity, coupled with proven clinical outcomes, positions ARMA as a cornerstone in the future of GERD management. With its potential to bridge the gap between pharmacological therapy and surgical intervention, ARMA offers a new hope for patients seeking relief from GERD.

Acknowledgments The author wishes to acknowledge the support of Showa University Koto Toyosu Hospital for providing access to clinical data and resources. Special thanks to the research team for their invaluable contributions. No external funding was used in the preparation of this chapter.

References

1. Eusebi LH, Ratnakumaran R, Yuan Y, Solaymani-Dodaran M, Bazzoli F, Ford AC. Global prevalence of, and risk factors for, gastro-oesophageal reflux symptoms: a meta-analysis. Gut. 2018;67(3):430–40.
2. El-Serag HB, Sweet S, Winchester CC, Dent J. Update on the epidemiology of gastro-oesophageal reflux disease: a systematic review. Gut. 2014;63(6):871–80.
3. Delshad SD, Almario CV, Chey WD, Spiegel BMR. Prevalence of gastroesophageal reflux disease and proton pump inhibitor-refractory symptoms. Gastroenterology. 2020;158(5):1250–61.e2.
4. Ito T, Jensen RT. Association of long-term proton pump inhibitor therapy with bone fractures and effects on absorption of calcium, vitamin B12, iron, and magnesium. Curr Gastroenterol Rep. 2010;12(6):448–57.
5. Testoni PA, Testoni S, Mazzoleni G, Vailati C, Passaretti S. Long-term efficacy of transoral incisionless fundoplication with Esophyx (Tif 2.0) and factors affecting outcomes in GERD patients followed for up to 6 years: a prospective single-center study. Surg Endosc. 2015;29(9):2770–80.
6. Kalapala R, Karyampudi A, Nabi Z, Darisetty S, Jagtap N, Ramchandani M, et al. Endoscopic full-thickness plication for the treatment of PPI-dependent GERD: results from a randomised, sham controlled trial. Gut. 2022;71(4):686–94.
7. Aziz AM, El-Khayat HR, Sadek A, Mattar SG, McNulty G, Kongkam P, et al. A prospective randomized trial of sham, single-dose Stretta, and double-dose Stretta for the treatment of gastroesophageal reflux disease. Surg Endosc. 2010;24(4):818–25.
8. Inoue H, Ito H, Ikeda H, Sato C, Sato H, Phalanusitthepha C, et al. Anti-reflux mucosectomy for gastroesophageal reflux disease in the absence of hiatus hernia: a pilot study. Ann Gastroenterol. 2014;27(4):346–51.
9. Sumi K, Inoue H, Kobayashi Y, Iwaya Y, Abad MRA, Fujiyoshi Y, et al. Endoscopic treatment of proton pump inhibitor-refractory gastroesophageal reflux disease with anti-reflux mucosectomy: experience of 109 cases. Dig Endosc. 2020;33:347.
10. Inoue H, Tanabe M, de Santiago ER, Abad MRA, Shimamura Y, Fujiyoshi Y, et al. Anti-reflux mucosal ablation (ARMA) as a new treatment for gastroesophageal reflux refractory to proton pump inhibitors: a pilot study. Endosc Int Open. 2020;8(2):E133–e8.
11. Shimamura Y, Inoue H, Tanabe M, Ushikubo K, Yamamoto K, Kimoto Y, et al. Clinical outcomes of anti-reflux mucosal ablation for gastroesophageal reflux disease: an international bi-institutional study. J Gastroenterol Hepatol. 2024;39(1):149–56.
12. Yeh JH, Lee CT, Hsu MH, Lin CW, Hsiao PJ, Chen CL, et al. Antireflux mucosal intervention (ARMI) procedures for refractory gastroesophageal reflux disease: a systematic review and meta-analysis. Ther Adv Gastroenterol. 2022;15:17562848221094959.
13. Rodríguez de Santiago E, Sanchez-Vegazo CT, Peñas B, Shimamura Y, Tanabe M, Álvarez-Díaz N, et al. Antireflux mucosectomy (ARMS) and antireflux mucosal ablation (ARMA) for gastroesophageal reflux disease: a systematic review and meta-analysis. Endosc Int Open. 2021;9(11):E1740–e51.

14. Inoue H, Yamamoto K, Shimamura Y, Azuma D, Ushikubo K, Okada H, et al. A pilot study on anti-reflux mucoplasty: advancing endoscopic anti-reflux therapy for gastro-esophageal reflux disease. Dig Endosc. 2023;36:690.
15. Inoue H, Yamamoto K, Tanaka I, Ushikubo K, Nishikawa Y, Sethi A, et al. Introducing antireflux mucoplasty with valve: a novel endoscopic treatment for GERD. VideoGIE. 2024;9(11):463–7.

Chapter 8
Transoral Incisionless Fundoplication (TIF)

Oscar A. Olavarria, Melissa M. Felinski, Shinil K. Shah, Erik B. Wilson, and Peter A. Walker

Background

- Transoral incisionless fundoplication (TIF) is a totally endoscopic technique utilized for the management of gastroesophageal reflux disease (GERD). TIF involves wrapping the fundus of the stomach 180°–300° posteriorly around the lower esophagus with the use of a specially designed flexible endoscopic tool. The objective of the TIF procedure is to restore the angle of His and create a new full thickness gastroesophageal valve which prevents gastric contents from refluxing back into the esophagus, thereby reducing symptoms and the potential complications of GERD.
- The EsophyX® (EndoGastric Solutions, Inc., Redmond, WA, United States) device, developed by Stefan Kraemer in 2003, was used to perform the first TIF procedure in 2005. Most of the initial clinical experience came from Europe and focused on the early versions of the device. The EsophyX® device was granted clearance by the United States Food and Drug Administration in 2007. However, during the early years of its introduction in the US market, the TIF procedure faced a lack of support as its precise role in managing GERD patients was still unclear. Several modifications have been made to the device to improve its performance, including the EsophyX2® and the newest iteration, the EsophyX Z®.
- TIF has gained popularity as a less invasive alternative to traditional surgical treatments for GERD with over 30,000 procedures completed. The American Medical Association has acknowledged the strong clinical evidence and created

O. A. Olavarria · M. M. Felinski · S. K. Shah · E. B. Wilson · P. A. Walker (✉)
Division of Minimally Invasive and Elective General Surgery, Department of Surgery, McGovern Medical School, University of Texas Health Science Center at Houston, Houston, TX, USA
e-mail: Oscar.A.Olavarria@uth.tmc.edu; Melissa.Felinski@uth.tmc.edu; Shinil.K.Shah@uth.tmc.edu; Erik.B.Wilson@uth.tmc.edu; peter.walker@uth.tmc.edu

M. Ujiki, Z. M. Callahan (eds.), *Third Space Endoscopy*,
https://doi.org/10.1007/978-3-031-84509-3_8

and implemented a unique category 1 code for the TIF procedure for the treatment of GERD.

Indications

- Transoral incisionless fundoplication with the EsophyX® device is approved for the treatment of chronic symptomatic GERD in patients who require and respond to pharmacological therapy such as proton pump inhibitors (PPIs) or H2 receptor antagonists. The TIF procedure also presents a viable alternative for patients who exhibit poor adherence to medication regimens, those who suffer from medication-induced side effects, or those who express a desire to discontinue their medical therapy. Additionally, TIF has been shown to be an effective treatment option for the repair of sliding hiatal hernias less than 2 cm in size in patients with symptomatic GERD as the device can reduce small hernias by advancing the endoscope caudally prior to deploying the fasteners during the creation of the fundoplication.
- There are several contraindications to the TIF procedure that should be taken into consideration. These include:
  - Inability to tolerate general anesthesia.
  - Esophageal ulcers, diverticula, or strictures.
  - Severe esophagitis.
  - Barrett's esophagus.
  - Esophageal motility disorders.
  - Peptic ulcer disease.
  - Hiatal hernia greater than 2 cm in size or paraesophageal hernia unless it will be repaired concomitantly.
  - Obesity with a body mass index (BMI) over 35 kg/m^2.
  - Pregnancy.
  - Immunosuppression.
  - Portal hypertension with esophageal varices, uncontrolled coagulopathy, or bleeding disorders.
  - Inability to comply with postoperative instructions including diet.
  - Although previous esophageal or gastric surgery are not absolute contraindications, patients with altered anatomy of these organs may not be ideal candidates for TIF.

Patient Evaluation

Initial Evaluation

- Optimal patient selection plays a crucial role in attaining favorable outcomes with antireflux procedures. In general, patients considered for a TIF should undergo a thorough evaluation starting with a detailed history with special emphasis on characterizing the typical and atypical GERD symptoms.
- While patients who exhibit good clinical response often desire to continue medical management, individuals with incomplete or limited response to PPI therapy may actively seek alternative treatment options. Moreover, for patients with more severe heartburn, preoperative counseling plays a crucial role in establishing realistic expectations including discussion of higher likelihood of needing additional acid suppression therapy alongside the TIF procedure to effectively manage GERD symptoms.

Diagnostic Studies

- Objective workup of patients suspected of having GERD include:
  - Barium esophagram looking for presence of hiatal hernia.
  - Esophagogastroduodenoscopy to grade the appearance of the antireflux barrier (Hill grade) and to confirm the absence of anatomical abnormalities or pathologies of the stomach and esophagus, including esophagitis and Barrett's esophagus.
  - Esophageal manometry study to rule out esophageal motility disorder.
  - pH probe study to quantify the degree of acid reflux which can be excluded in the presence of severe (Los Angeles grade C or D) esophagitis,
- Traditionally, patients with an abnormal 24-h pH score, patients with typical GERD symptoms, and patients who experience improvement of symptoms with PPI therapy have experienced the most successful outcomes following antireflux procedures. Optimal TIF outcomes are more probable when there is minimal structural deterioration of the gastroesophageal flap valve as represented by a low-grade Hill classification [1].

Technique

Planning

- The majority of TIF procedures are performed in an operating room or in an appropriately equipped endoscopy facility.
- Patients are initially placed in supine position for the induction of general endotracheal anesthesia. At some institutions, patients will be nasotracheally intubated to allow for the oropharynx to be used entirely for the TIF device.

Endoscopic Access and Anatomical Landmarks

- After intubation, the patient may be placed in partial left lateral decubitus.
- Prior to the procedure, an esophagogastroduodenoscopy with a conventional endoscope is performed to verify the anatomic landmarks.
- The esophagus can then be dilated with the use of a large bore bougie in order to facilitate the advancement of the TIF device into the stomach. It is optional to introduce an overtube to protect against mucosal damage, yet, if no overtube is inserted, then a bite block should be placed to protect the teeth.

Procedure (Esophyx®)

- The EsophyX® (EndoGastric Solutions, Inc.) is a disposable, 57 French, flexible, multichannel endoluminal device. A conventional endoscope is introduced through one of the channels down the center of the device and provides visualization of the procedure at all times. The rest of the channels are for surgical instruments.
- Typically, two proceduralists are needed to perform the procedure: one experienced endoscopist who operates the EsophyX® device and an assistant to operate the endoscope.
- After lubricating the device, it is inserted through the patient's mouth into the esophagus and stomach under direct visualization. Once inside of the stomach, insufflation is completed with carbon dioxide. After visualizing the articulating arm, the endoscope is retracted into the body of the device, the articulating arm is flexed, and the endoscope is again advanced and retroflexed to place the gastroesophageal junction (GEJ) in view (Fig. 8.1). The GEJ view is conventionally oriented in a clock face fashion with the 12-o'clock position resembling the lesser curvature and the greater curvature at the 6-o'clock position.
- The helix retractor is introduced into the GEJ at the 12-o'clock position, and tissue is then pulled into the jaws of the articulating arm. Subsequently, the entire

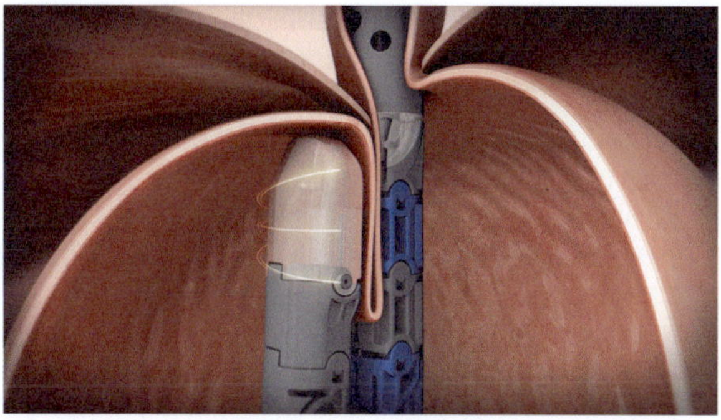

Fig. 8.1 Schematic representation of transoral incisionless fundoplication with the EsophyX® device. (Image courtesy of EndoGastric Solutions, Inc.)

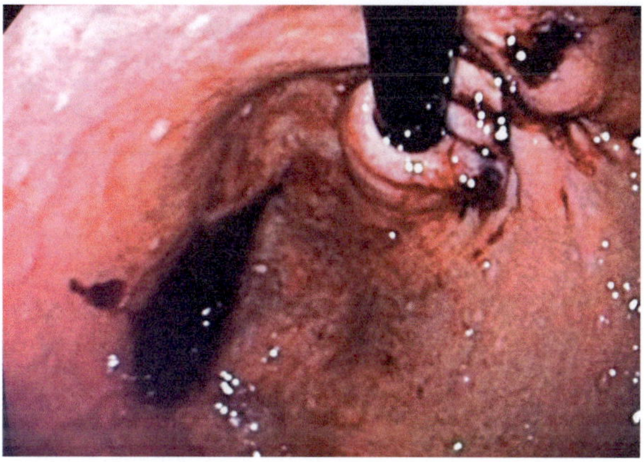

Fig. 8.2 Endoscopic view of new flap valve after transoral incisionless fundoplication with the EsophyX® device

device is advanced distally 2–3 cm to ensure that any small sliding hiatal hernia is reduced and also ensure that the targeted tissue for fixation is below the diaphragm. A series of SerosaFuse® "H"-shaped polypropylene fasteners are deployed by a trigger mechanism operated by the endoscopist to create serosa-to-serosa plications. These steps are serially repeated deploying around 12–20 fasteners in order to accomplish a circumferential 180°–300° wrap around the GEJ (Fig. 8.2).

- After completion, the EsophyX® device is completely withdrawn, and the conventional endoscope is again introduced to evaluate the new fundoplication as well as assess for bleeding or injuries.

Procedure (MUSE™)

- The Medigus Ultrasonic Surgical Endostapler or MUSE™ (Medigus Ltd., Omer, Israel) system is a disposable, single-use, flexible endoluminal device also utilized for the creation of an endoscopic fundoplication. The device is equipped with a high-definition micro video camera, illumination, and an ultrasonic range finder which is used to measure the thickness and degree of compression of tissue between the sensor and its receiver on the shaft.

- As opposed to the EsophyX® device which deploys fasteners, the MUSE™ differs in that it staples. The shaft of the device contains the staple cartridge with a total of 5 B-shaped 4.8 mm titanium staples, and the tip of the endoscope has the anvil to bend the staples.
- In general, one endoscopist is sufficient to perform the procedure.
- The device is introduced through the mouth, advanced into the stomach, and retroflexed to place the GEJ into view. After selecting the stapling site, the device is pulled back to set the stapling cartridge approximately 3 cm above the GEJ. The tip of the device is then bent to clamp the tissue. The anvil screws are deployed, the tissue is compressed to 1.4–1.6 mm, and the staples are then fired. The anvil screws are retrieved, the scope is straightened, and the endostapler is withdrawn. These steps are repeated circumferentially around the GEJ to create a new 180°–300° flap valve.

Postoperative Care

- TIF is typically performed on an outpatient basis and requires only a short recovery period. Patients can usually return home on the same day and resume normal activities within a few days.
- In general, patients are asked to follow dietary restrictions after the procedure which include a liquid diet for approximately 2 weeks prior to progressing to soft diet and then regular diet.
- Patients are asked to avoid strenuous activities for the immediate perioperative period. Finally, patients are asked to continue their PPIs for several weeks to allow for healing of the gastric mucosa.

Outcomes

- A significant amount of controversy exists around the definition of efficacy and effectiveness of therapies aimed at the management of GERD. There are multiple endpoints that can be used to assess treatment effect including normalization of pH, improvement of typical or atypical symptoms, cessation of PPI use, improvement in esophagitis, or improvement in quality of life (QOL). Moreover, studies have failed to find associations between resolution of abnormal esophageal acid exposure and symptom improvement after interventions for GERD [2]. The lack of consensus on which endpoints to use therefore results in difficult comparisons of the data across the published literature.

EsophyX®

- The TEMPO study compared TIF with maximal dose PPI in patients with less than a 2 cm hiatal hernia and demonstrated heartburn was eliminated in 90% of patients randomized to TIF and only in 13% of patients randomized to PPI [3]. Moreover, regurgitation and extraesophageal symptoms were eliminated in 62% patients undergoing TIF and 5% in the PPI group. Interestingly, no significant difference was found in the rate of abnormal esophageal acid exposure. At 6 months, all patients crossed over to TIF, and symptoms were eliminated in 88% at 3 years and in 80% of patients at 5 years [4, 5] Similarly, regurgitation was eliminated in 90% (37/41) and 86% of patients (37/43) at 3 and 5 years, respectively. Complete cessation of PPI was only achieved in 46% (20/44) of patients who completed follow-up (34% were taking daily PPI and 20% were occasionally using PPI). No significant serious adverse events were observed during this period. Authors therefore concluded that TIF is safe, effective, and durable for the management of GERD in selected patients.
- Another landmark publication is the Randomized EsophyX® vs. Sham, Placebo-Controlled Transoral Fundoplication (RESPECT) trial [6]. This was a multicenter study, conducted at eight centers in the United States. The patient population was similar to that of the TEMPO trial. Enrolled patients had GERD symptoms and troublesome regurgitation refractory to PPI therapy for at least 6 months and abnormal pH testing. Patients with any of the previously mentioned contraindications for TIF with the EsophyX2® device were excluded from the study. A total of 129 patients were enrolled and randomized in a 2:1 ratio: 87 to TIF with the EsophyX2® device + placebo (intervention group) versus 42 patients randomized to sham endoscopy with esophageal dilation under general anesthesia + PPI therapy (control group). The primary outcome was the proportion of patients who had elimination of troublesome regurgitation. At 6-month follow-up, 67% (58/87) of TIF/placebo patients reported elimination of regurgitation vs. 45% (19/42) in patients in the sham/PPI group (RR = 1.47, 95% CI = 1.02–2.12, P = 0.02). Moreover, at 3-month follow-up, 11% of patients in the TIF/placebo group experienced early treatment failure defined as persistent and troublesome symptoms versus 36% in the sham/PPI group (RR = 0.32, 95% CI = 0.15–0.65, P < 0.01). Additionally, patients who underwent the TIF procedure demonstrated significant decreases in esophageal acid exposure in all measured parameters including mean number of reflux episodes (135 before TF to 94 after TF, P < 0.01), mean percent total time under pH of 4 (9.3 before TF to 6.4 after TF, P < 0.01), and DeMeester scores (33.6 before TF to 23.9 after TF, P < 0.01). There was no significant improvement in pH control among patients randomized to the sham/PPI group. Finally, among the patients in the TIF/placebo group who had esophagitis on screening and underwent endoscopy at 6 months, esophagitis was healed in 77% versus 50% in the sham/PPI group.
- It is important to note that the excellent clinical outcomes observed in the TEMPO study can be partially attributed to patient selection that included

patients with Hill grades I and II while excluding those with severe erosive esophagitis (Los Angeles grade C or D). In contrast, the slightly lower rates of resolution of bothersome GERD symptoms observed in the RESPECT trial can be attributed to the inclusion of patients with Hill grade III and more advanced disease.

- Another important multicenter randomized controlled trial was a study conducted in Europe on a similar patient population and published by Håkansson et al. [7]. This study randomized 44 patients to TIF with the EsophyX2 device versus a sham endoscopy without PPI. The primary endpoint was the time to "treatment failure" defined as a composite of need for PPI, persistent heartburn, regurgitation or dysphagia for 7 days, persistent esophagitis, or reinterventions. Authors found a significant difference in remission which favored patients undergoing TIF (mean days to remission, 197 vs. 107, $P < 0.01$). Moreover, patients who underwent TIF had significant improvement in quality of life where those treated with PPI experienced no improvement. After 6 months of follow-up, the percentage of patients who were able to discontinue daily PPI was significantly higher in the TIF group (59%) compared to the sham group (18%) ($P = 0.01$). Finally, the percentage of patients with normalized esophageal acid exposure was much higher in the TIF group (69%) than in the control group (20%) ($P < 0.01$).
- Currently, there is a lack of studies with direct comparison of the safety and effectiveness of the TIF procedure versus other surgical treatments such as Nissen or Toupet fundoplication. However, several studies have made indirect comparisons through meta-analyses of published evidence including a large network meta-analysis published in 2018 by Richter et al. [8]. Authors included 7 RCTs with nearly 1200 patients; 2 studies compared TIF to PPI, 2 compared TIF to sham, and 3 compared Nissen to PPI. The study found that Nissen was superior to TIF for the percentage of time with pH <4 (OR = 0.08, 95% CI = 0.02–0.36, $P < 0.01$). Additionally, authors found that, based on Bayesian analysis, Nissen fundoplication had the highest probability of increasing LES pressure and resolving esophagitis. Interestingly, TIF had the highest probability of improving QOL.
- This study has been, however, heavily criticized for multiple reasons. First, conclusions which presented Nissen as a superior alternative were made based on indirect evidence. Moreover, the only outcome with a significant difference had an odds ratio of 0.08, which seems extreme and difficult to believe. Additionally, the degree of statistical and clinical heterogeneity was extremely high with TIF studies having mild esophagitis, small hiatal hernias (<2 cm), varying baseline responsiveness to PPIs, and lower esophagitis grade. Furthermore, they included TIF studies with different iterations of the device and the procedure (TIF v1 and TIF v2). Also, the authors claimed that the trend in superiority of TIF for improving QOL is confounded by the short duration of follow-up, yet they did not include the 3-year follow-up of the TEMPO trial which was already published at that time. Finally, the authors chose primary outcomes different from those of the included trials, instead, focusing on primary outcomes that readily place Nissen

fundoplication at an advantage compared with the other two interventions (i.e., there is no biological plausibility for PPIs to impact LES pressures).

Concomitant Transoral Incisionless Fundoplication (cTIF)

- Another novel technique is the concomitant transoral incisionless fundoplication (cTIF) which combines laparoscopic hiatal hernia repair and TIF into a single-stage intervention. (Fig. 8.3). This approach is intended for patients who have hiatal hernias exceeding 2 cm in which performing a TIF alone is highly likely to fail. Supporters of cTIF assert that TIF offers several advantages. Firstly, it establishes a flap valve at the gastric cardia while preserving the fundus, which

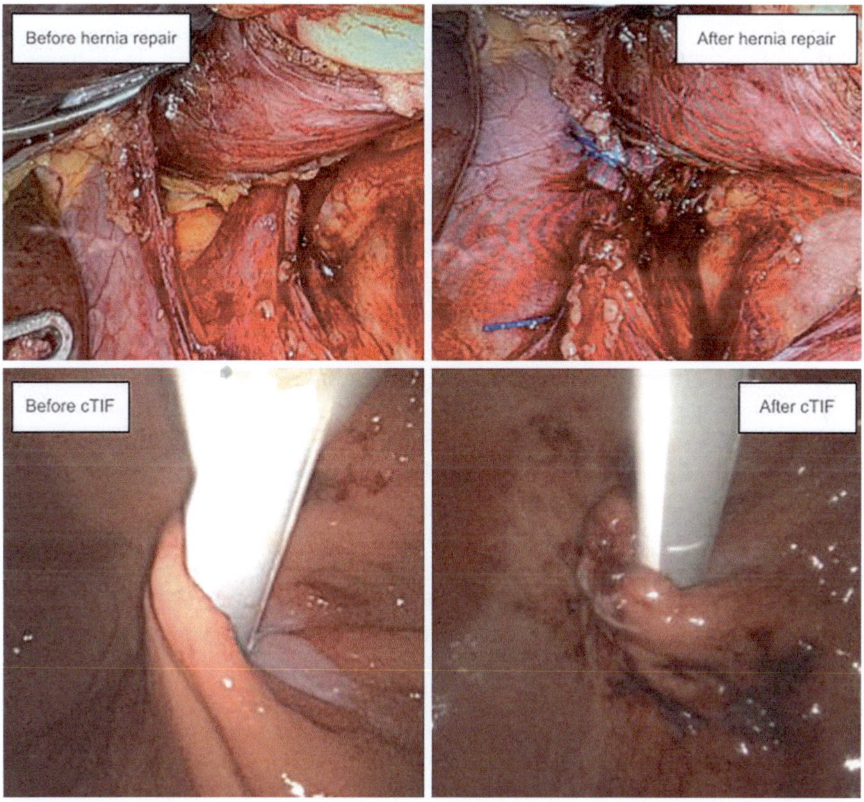

Fig. 8.3 Endoscopic and laparoscopic view before and after concomitant transoral incisionless fundoplication (cTIF)

is advantageous for future revisional surgery, particularly in young patients. Secondly, it reduces the likelihood of gas bloat. Additionally, the standardization of the wrap allows for comparability across various studies of cTIF. Currently, there are no published RCT studies on this topic, and the current evidence is limited to observational studies.

- In 2019, Janu et al. published a case series of 90 patients who underwent cTIF [9]. Enrolled patients had moderate to severe GERD symptoms for over 1 year, had a partial or complete response to PPI after at least 6 months of medical therapy, and had a hiatal hernia between 2 and 5 cm on endoscopy. The primary focus was to assess the efficacy of cTIF in terms of symptom control and improvement in quality of life. Authors demonstrated that cTIF resulted in significant improvement in heartburn, regurgitation, and dysphagia, in addition to significant improvements in quality of life for patients with GERD. Moreover, the majority of patients were able to discontinue their use of PPI (70% and 74% of patients were off PPI at 6 months and 1 year, respectively). The procedure was found to be safe with no reported postoperative complications, and reportedly, no patient complained of experiencing gas bloat, inability to belch, or inability to vomit following the procedure. The main limitations of this study are the lack of a comparison group and the lack of long-term follow-up.
- Another case series was published by Choi et al. in 2021 [10]. This series included 60 patients who underwent cTIF at a single institution. Authors enrolled patients with significant GERD (Barrett's esophagus, Los Angeles grade C or D esophagitis, or a DeMeester score > 14.7 on pH testing) and with a hiatal hernia >2 cm in size or Hill grade valve >2. Following the cTIF procedure, significant improvement in symptoms were observed across all quality-of-life questionnaires. Additionally, mean DeMeester scores decreased from 43.7 preoperatively to 4.9 after cTIF, and esophageal acid exposure time decreased from 12.7% to 1.28%, respectively. One serious intraoperative adverse event was reported consisting of an esophageal mucosal injury which was successfully managed by closing the defect using four endoscopic hemoclips.
- In 2023, Jaruvongvanich et al. published a multicenter retrospective cohort study of cTIF versus laparoscopic hiatal hernia repair plus Nissen fundoplication [11]. This study included a total of 195 patients, 125 patients who underwent cTIF, and 70 patients who underwent hiatal hernia repair along with Nissen fundoplication. Their primary endpoint was the incidence of adverse events defined as Clavien-Dindo complications grades III–V. Authors found a lower incidence of early serious adverse events (0% vs. 4.3%, $P < 0.01$) as well as lower incidence of early nonserious adverse events within 30 days postop in the TIF group (0% vs. 18.6%, $P < 0.01$). There were no statistically significant differences in rates of reflux symptom-free off PPI (60.8% vs. 62.9%, $P = 0.78$ at 6 months and 52.5% vs. 58.1%, $P = 0.53$ at 12 months), rates of dysphagia (8.3% vs. 14.3%, $P = 0.10$ at 6 months and 10.1% vs. 12.9%, $P = 0.62$ at 12 months), or PPI discontinuation (73.8% vs. 60.6%, $P = 0.07$ at 6 months and 73.5% vs. 58.3%, $P = 0.07$ at 12 months). The TIF group had a significantly lower rate of gas bloating at 6 months (13.8% vs. 30.0%, $P < 0.01$), shorter hospital stay (1 [IQR 1–2]

days vs. 2 [IQR 1–2] days, $P < 0.01$), and a lower 30-day readmission rate (0% vs. 4.3%, $P = 0.01$).

MUSE™

- To this day, no randomized trials have been carried out evaluating patient outcomes with the use of this device, and the data that is published is scarce and mostly represented by observational studies. The first publication on the long-term outcomes of the MUSE™ device was published by Roy-Shapira et al. [12]. They enrolled 13 adult patients with GERD who had incomplete response to PPI and who were found to have abnormal 24-hour pH test or esophagitis. Authors were able to achieve 85% (11/13 patients) follow-up at 5 years. The primary outcome was the proportion of patients with at least 50% improvement in quality-of-life scores off PPI assessed through the GERD-HRQL; this was achieved by 92% (12/13) of patients. At 5 years, 64% (7/13) of patients were off PPIs, and another 23% (3/13) reduced their PPI use by at least 50%.
- In 2015, Zacherl et al. published the early results of a prospective multicenter case series [13]. The study was conducted in six institutions across Europe, India, and the United States. Authors enrolled adult patients with at least 2 years of GERD symptoms, who had pathologic reflux confirmed on pH monitoring test off PPI and who had at least 6 months use of PPI. Exclusion criteria were similar to those of the EsophyX® device. Similar to the pilot study by Roy-Shapira et al., their primary endpoint was the proportion of patients with at least 50% improvement in GERD-HRQL scores off PPI. A total of 66 patients were included in the analysis. At the 6-month follow-up, a minimum of 50% improvement in GERD-HRQL scores were observed in 73% (48/66) of patients. Additionally, 64.6% (42/66) of patients were no longer taking daily PPIs at 6 months. A significant improvement in several esophageal acid exposure parameters was found including less total number of reflux episodes and lower percent total time and upright time with pH less than 4. There were two serious adverse events: one patient developed an esophageal leak requiring antibiotics and chest tube placement, and the other patient had a gastrointestinal bleed requiring endoscopy and transfusions. Kim et al. published the 4-year follow-up results on the same cohort of patients presented in the paper by Zacherl et al. [14]. This long term follow-up study was importantly limited by the fact that only 56% (37/66) of patients completed follow-up, as data was only able to be obtained from three of the six enrolling centers. Among the patients who completed the follow-up, there was a notable improvement in their GERD-HRQL scores from a median of 29.1 at baseline to 5.3 at 4 years post-intervention. Additionally, 69.4% remained off daily PPI.
- Another single-center case series was published by Testoni et al. in 2022 [15]. They enrolled 45 adult patients with chronic symptomatic GERD who had partial or complete response to PPIs, who underwent endoluminal fundoplication

with the MUSE™ device and prospectively followed them for 3 years. Their primary outcome was the percentage of patients who stopped or halved their PPI use. At 6 months post-intervention, esophageal acid exposure improved in nearly half of patients. Authors were able to achieve 71% follow-up at 3 years. Based on intention-to-treat analysis, 77% of patients completely stopped taking or halved their PPI dose intake. Quality of life scores as measured by GERD-HRQL and RSI questionnaires were significantly improved after endoluminal fundoplication with the MUSE™ device. At the 3-year follow-up, 60% of patients indicated at least a 50% improvement of quality of life with the procedure. Authors reported two major complications which required surgical repair: one intraoperative gastric perforation and one delayed esophageal perforation. Finally, one additional patient was unresponsive to endoluminal fundoplication by the MUSE™ device and underwent Nissen fundoplication within 6 months after the procedure.

Pearls	Pitfalls
Insertion of device	Begin by performing an esophagogastroduodenoscopy. Recommend use of CO_2 insufflation during the entire procedure to reduce abdominal distension and pain Mount the device over the conventional endoscopy Guide the endoscope all the way into the stomach and with the endoscope in place, and carefully guide the device down into the esophagus through a Seldinger technique Do not force the advancement of the device. If there is resistance at the soft palate, guide the device with the use of your fingers. If there is resistance at the pharynx, consider deflating the balloon of the endotracheal tube
Positioning of device	Once the device is advanced into the stomach, confirm appropriate insufflation of the stomach to avoid scraping of the mucosa by the device Rotate the device to align it with the greater curvature of the stomach to also avoid scraping of the mucosa and therefore prevent bleeding Subsequently, pull back the endoscope to allow articulation of the flexible end of the device Advance the endoscope and retroflex to visualize the hiatus
Creation of flap valve	Begin with a suture pattern at the corners and progress by building rotation. Build height along the greater curvature, at least 3 cm Use all points of retraction which include the helix retractor which pulls the GEJ into the jaw of the device, the anvil at the tip of the device which manipulates the fundus and cardia of the stomach, and the suction system which retracts the esophagus to allow reduction of the prolapsed GEJ into the abdomen. This allows for less diaphragm incorporation into the fasteners once fired Patients with more laxity of phrenoesophageal ligament will allow for better reduction of the stomach and GEJ complex off the diaphragm Pull as much tissue depth as possible into the device while advancing the device the farthest possible from the hiatus
Deployment of fasteners	Visualize each fastener to confirm appropriate loading prior to firing of the device In the event of a misfire of a fastener, refire into free space and clear the sutures out to avoid reloading of fasteners on top of previously misfired fasteners

(continued)

Pearls	Pitfalls
Retrieval of device	Pull back the endoscope before straightening the device After straightening the device, push the endoscope back down and remove the entire device in line Confirm the helix retractor is in the appropriate position before removal of the device to avoid scraping of the mucosa or potential perforation

References

1. Testoni PA, Testoni S, Mazzoleni G, Vailati C, Passaretti S. Long-term efficacy of transoral incisionless fundoplication with Esophyx (Tif 2.0) and factors affecting outcomes in GERD patients followed for up to 6 years: a prospective single-center study. Surg Endosc. 2015;29(9):2770–80. Available from: https://link.springer.com/article/10.1007/s00464-014-4008-6
2. Milkes D, Gerson LB, Triadafilopoulos G. Complete elimination of reflux symptoms does not guarantee normalization of intraesophageal and intragastric pH in patients with gastroesophageal reflux disease (GERD). Am J Gastroenterol. 2004;99(6):991–6. Available from: https://pubmed.ncbi.nlm.nih.gov/15180715/
3. Trad KS, Barnes WE, Simoni G, Shughoury AB, Mavrelis PG, Raza M, et al. Transoral incisionless fundoplication effective in eliminating GERD symptoms in partial responders to proton pump inhibitor therapy at 6 months: the TEMPO randomized clinical trial. Surg Innov. 2015;22(1):26.
4. Trad KS, Fox MA, Simoni G, Shughoury AB, Mavrelis PG, Raza M, et al. Transoral fundoplication offers durable symptom control for chronic GERD: 3-year report from the TEMPO randomized trial with a crossover arm. Surg Endosc. 2017;31(6):2498.
5. Trad KS, Barnes WE, Prevou ER, Simoni G, Steffen JA, Shughoury AB, et al. The TEMPO trial at 5 years: transoral fundoplication (TIF 2.0) is safe, durable, and cost-effective. Surg Innov. 2018;25(2):149–57. Available from: https://pubmed.ncbi.nlm.nih.gov/29405886/
6. Hunter JG, Kahrilas PJ, Bell RCW, Wilson EB, Trad KS, Dolan JP, et al. Efficacy of transoral fundoplication vs omeprazole for treatment of regurgitation in a randomized controlled trial. Gastroenterology. 2015;148(2):324–33. Available from: https://pubmed.ncbi.nlm.nih.gov/25448925/
7. Montgomery M, Cadiere GB, Rajan A, Bruley Des Varannes S, Lerhun M, Coron E, et al. Randomised clinical trial: transoral incisionless fundoplication vs. sham intervention to control chronic GERD. Aliment Pharmacol Ther. 2015;42(11–12):1261–70. Available from: https://pubmed.ncbi.nlm.nih.gov/26463242/
8. Richter JE, Kumar A, Lipka S, Miladinovic B, Velanovich V. Efficacy of laparoscopic Nissen fundoplication vs Transoral incisionless fundoplication or proton pump inhibitors in patients with gastroesophageal reflux disease: a systematic review and network meta-analysis. Gastroenterology. 2018;154(5):1298–308. Available from: https://pubmed.ncbi.nlm.nih.gov/29305934/
9. Janu P, Shughoury AB, Venkat K, Hurwich D, Galouzis T, Siatras J, et al. Laparoscopic hiatal hernia repair followed by transoral incisionless fundoplication with EsophyX device (HH + TIF): efficacy and safety in two community hospitals. Surg Innov. 2019;26(6):675–86. Available from: https://pubmed.ncbi.nlm.nih.gov/31431138/
10. Choi AY, Roccato MK, Samarasena JB, Kolb JM, Lee DP, Lee RH, et al. Novel interdisciplinary approach to GERD: concomitant laparoscopic hiatal hernia repair with transoral incisionless fundoplication. J Am Coll Surg. 2021;232(3):309–18. Available from: https://journals.lww.com/journalacs/fulltext/2021/03000/novel_interdisciplinary_approach_to_gerd_.12.aspx

11. Jaruvongvanich VK, Matar R, Reisenauer J, Janu P, Mavrelis P, Ihde G, et al. Hiatal hernia repair with transoral incisionless fundoplication versus Nissen fundoplication for gastroesophageal reflux disease: a retrospective study. Endosc Int Open. 2023;11(1):E11.
12. Roy-Shapira A, Bapaye A, Date S, Pujari R, Dorwat S. Trans-oral anterior fundoplication: 5-year follow-up of pilot study. Surg Endosc. 2015;29(12):3717.
13. Zacherl J, Roy-Shapira A, Bonavina L, Bapaye A, Kiesslich R, Schoppmann SF, et al. Endoscopic anterior fundoplication with the Medigus Ultrasonic Surgical Endostapler (MUSE™) for gastroesophageal reflux disease: 6-month results from a multi-center prospective trial. Surg Endosc. 2015;29(1):220.
14. Kim HJ, Il KC, Kessler WR, Selzer DJ, McNulty G, Bapaye A, et al. Long-term follow-up results of endoscopic treatment of gastroesophageal reflux disease with the MUSE™ endoscopic stapling device. Surg Endosc. 2016;30(8):3402–8. Available from: https://pubmed.ncbi.nlm.nih.gov/26537905/
15. Testoni SGG, Cilona MB, Mazzoleni G, Fanti L, Ribichini E, Cavestro GM, et al. Transoral incisionless fundoplication with Medigus ultrasonic surgical endostapler (MUSE) for the treatment of gastro-esophageal reflux disease: outcomes up to 3 years. Surg Endosc. 2022;36(7):5023–31. Available from: https://link.springer.com/article/10.1007/s00464-021-08860-w

Part III
Muscle Division

Chapter 9
Peroral Endoscopic Myotomy (POEM)

Andrew Kastenmeier

Background

- The first reported cardioesophageal myotomy for achalasia was performed by Ernst Heller on April 14, 1913, at the University of Leipzig in Germany [1]. The patient was a 49-year-old man with idiopathic achalasia.
- In 1980, the first report of an endoscopic myotomy for the treatment of achalasia was published [2]. Seventeen patients with achalasia in Caracas, Venezuela, underwent endoscopic incision of the mucosa and circular muscle fibers for a short segment near the gastroesophageal junction. The authors reported good clinical results for patients at 25 months follow-up; however, this technique did not gain traction and no other reports were produced.
- In the early 2000s, great interest developed in what became termed natural orifice transluminal endoscopic surgery (NOTES). To facilitate NOTES, work was done to develop safe methods for endoscopic entry into the mediastinum, thoracic cavity, and peritoneal cavity. Solutions emerged including descriptions of creating a submucosal tunnel within the esophageal wall before entering the mediastinal cavity. This tunnel would create offsetting defects within the esophageal mucosa and the esophageal muscularis. This approach was termed the submucosal endoscopy with mucosal flap (SEMF) technique [3].
- In 2007, Jay Pasricha and colleagues reported the first *submucosal endoscopic esophageal myotomy* [4]. The procedure was performed in four pigs. All animals survived the procedure without complication, and postoperative manometry revealed a significant reduction in average LES pressure. There was no evidence of mediastinitis on necropsy.

A. Kastenmeier (✉)
Department of Surgery, Medical College of Wisconsin, Milwaukee, WI, USA
e-mail: akastenm@mcw.edu

M. Ujiki, Z. M. Callahan (eds.), *Third Space Endoscopy*,
https://doi.org/10.1007/978-3-031-84509-3_9

- Just 2 years later, Dr. Haruhiro Inoue and colleagues reported the first series of patients undergoing a submucosal endoscopic myotomy for achalasia [5]. In this manuscript, the term *per oral endoscopic myotomy or POEM* was introduced and has become the standard name for this procedure.
- Since 2010, POEM has become one of the most widely applied third space endoscopic techniques. POEM is now accepted as an equivalent to a laparoscopic Heller myotomy in terms of safety and efficacy, and in some cases, POEM is considered the preferred approach over laparoscopic Heller myotomy.

Indications

- POEM is indicated for the treatment of idiopathic achalasia; types I, II, and III [6–8]; and achalasia in the setting of Chagas disease. POEM and laparoscopic Heller myotomy are considered the most effective and durable treatments for achalasia type I and achalasia type II, whereas POEM is considered the most effective and durable treatment for achalasia type III.
- POEM is also indicated for the treatment of patients with persistent or recurrent esophageal outflow obstruction secondary to achalasia after a prior myotomy.
- There is emerging data suggesting that POEM is a treatment option for selected spastic motility disorders of the esophagus including esophagogastric junction outflow obstruction (EGJOO), hypercontractile esophagus, and distal esophageal spasm (DES).

Patient Evaluation

Initial Evaluation

- A thorough history and physical should be performed with a particular emphasis on duration and severity of symptoms as well as risk factors for esophageal cancer.
- Every patient should have a reported Eckhardt score (Table 9.1). This provides a baseline symptom measurement using a validated objective tool.

Table 9.1 Eckardt score for Achalasia symptom severity

Dysphagia	Regurgitation	Retrosternal chest pain	Weight loss	Score
None	None	None	None	0
Occasional	Occasional	Occasional	< 5 kg	1
Daily	Daily	Daily	5–10 kg	2
With each meal	With each meal	With each meal	> 10 kg	3

Diagnostic Studies

- High-resolution manometry is the gold standard test for definitive diagnosis of achalasia (Fig. 9.1). The Chicago Classification provides manometric diagnostic criteria for achalasia [9]. The Chicago Classification provides diagnostic criteria which also allows determination of achalasia subtype (Table 9.2). Differentiation of achalasia subtype aids in determining the prognosis and treatment options.
- According to the Chicago Classification, manometric criteria for type I achalasia, known as "classic achalasia," include 100% failed peristalsis and elevated integrated relaxation pressure (IRP) at the gastroesophageal junction (Fig. 9.2).

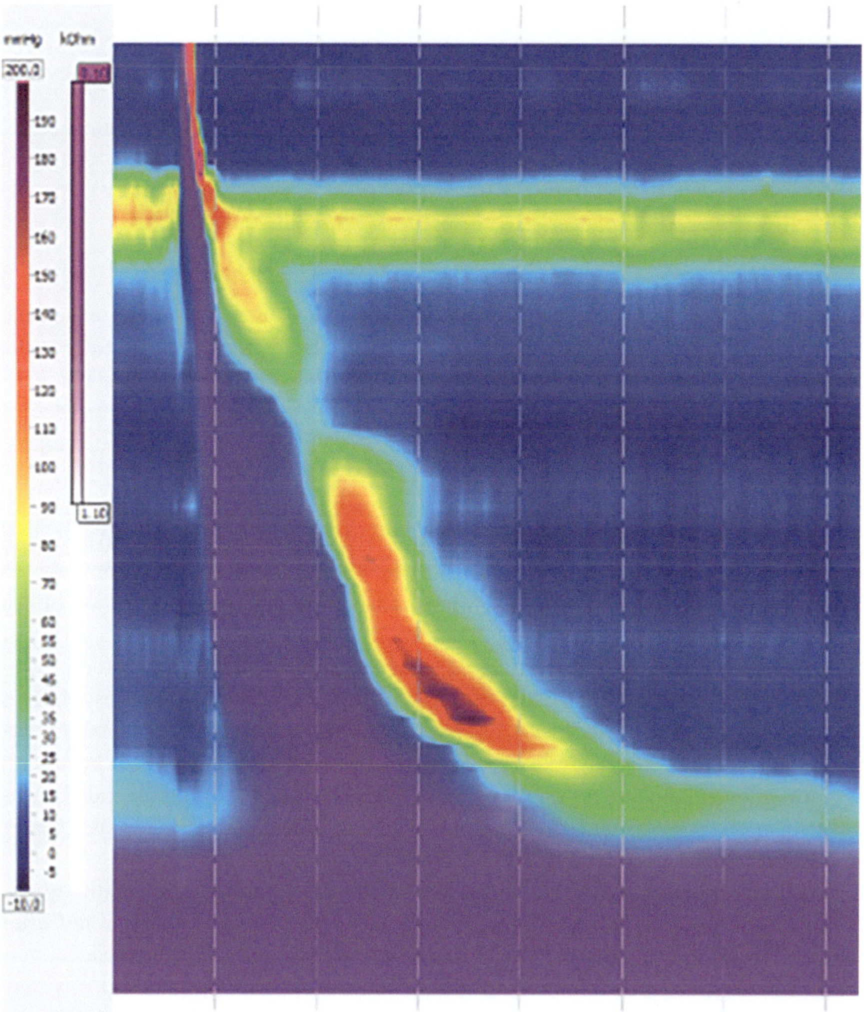

Fig. 9.1 High-resolution manometry without abnormality

Table 9.2 Chicago Classification v4.0 for achalasia subtypes and spastic esophageal motility disorders

Motility disorder	High resolution manometry diagnostic criteria
Achalasia, type I	100% failed peristalsis Elevated median IRP
Achalasia, type II	100% failed peristalsis Elevated median IRP Panesophageal pressurization in ≥20% of swallows
Achalasia, type III	No normal peristalsis Elevated median IRP Premature (spastic) esophageal contractions in ≥20% of swallows
Esophagogastric junction outflow obstruction (EGJOO)	Normal peristalsis Elevated median IRP Elevated intrabolus pressure
Distal esophageal spasm (DES)	Normal IRP Premature (spastic) contraction in ≥20% of swallows
Hypercontractile esophagus	Normal IRP Hypercontractile in ≥20% of swallows

IRP integrated relaxation pressure

Manometric criteria for type II achalasia, the most common form of achalasia, also includes 100% failed peristalsis and an elevated IRP but also requires the presence of pan pressurization of the esophagus in ≥20% of swallows (Fig. 9.3). Type III achalasia, known as "spastic achalasia," is defined by an absence of normal peristalsis, an elevated IRP, and episodes of premature (spastic) esophageal contractions in ≥20% of swallows (Fig. 9.4).

- Although a contrast esophagram is not adequate to definitively make the diagnosis of achalasia, this test remains an essential aspect of the preoperative evaluation. A timed barium esophagram is the most helpful version of this test as patients with achalasia will often have a standing column of contrast in the esophagus with delayed passage of contrast into the stomach, smooth tapering of the distal esophagus with relative esophageal outflow obstruction at the gastroesophageal junction (GEJ), and esophageal dilation with or without esophageal tortuosity (Fig. 9.5). Additionally, esophagram provides information about alternative or coexisting pathology that may impact the recommended treatment. Examples of findings on esophagram that that may impact recommended treatment include epiphrenic diverticulum (Fig. 9.6), Zenker's diverticulum, paraesophageal hernia, or abnormalities consistent with a tumor.
- Esophagram can provide prognostic information as well. Patients with significant esophageal dilation and/or tortuosity may have less symptom relief after treatment (Fig. 9.7). Despite a successful myotomy to relieve the esophageal outflow obstruction, patients with significant esophageal dilation and tortuosity may still experience dysphagia and regurgitation secondary to stasis within the

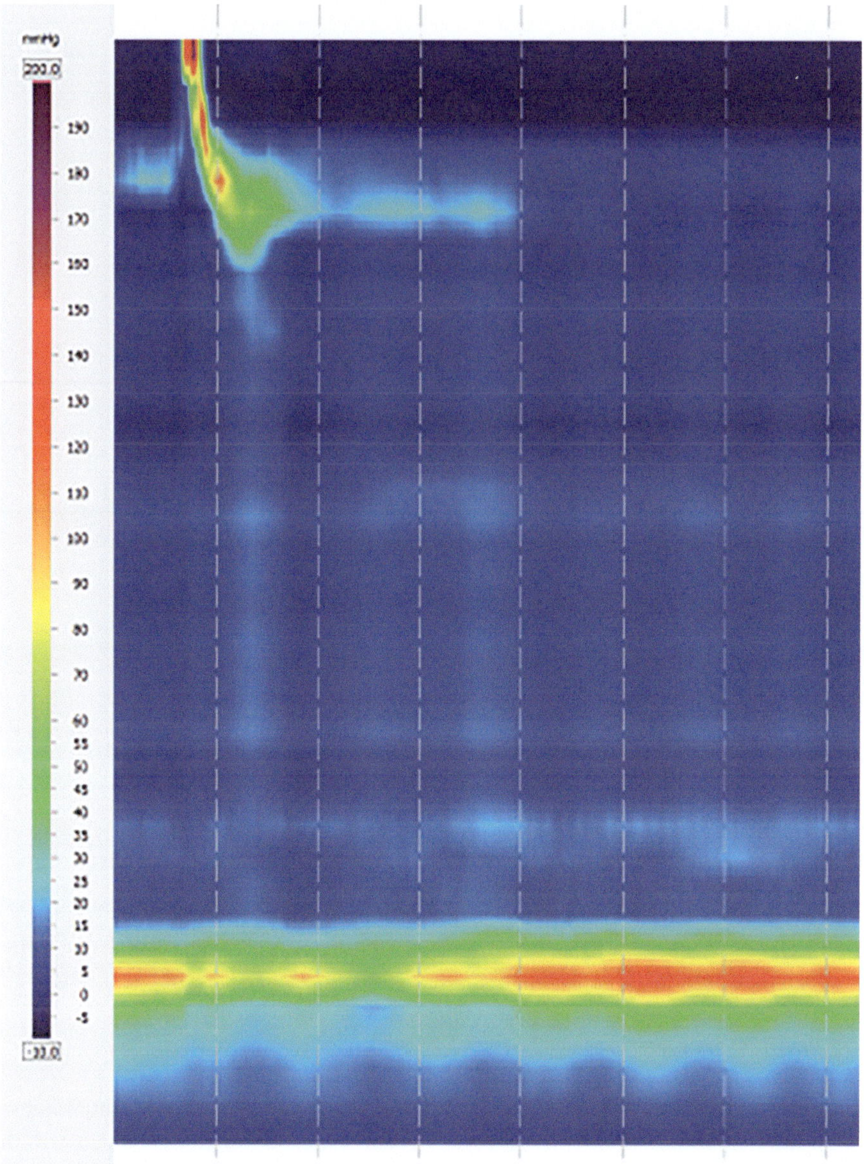

Fig. 9.2 High-resolution manometry showing achalasia, type I

dilated, horizontal aspects of the esophagus. This test also provides a baseline functional assessment in the event postoperative comparisons are necessary.

- Esophagogastroduodenoscopy (EGD) does not adequately make the diagnosis of achalasia; however, this test remains an essential aspect of the preoperative evaluation. Patients with achalasia may have a dilated or tortuous esophagus with

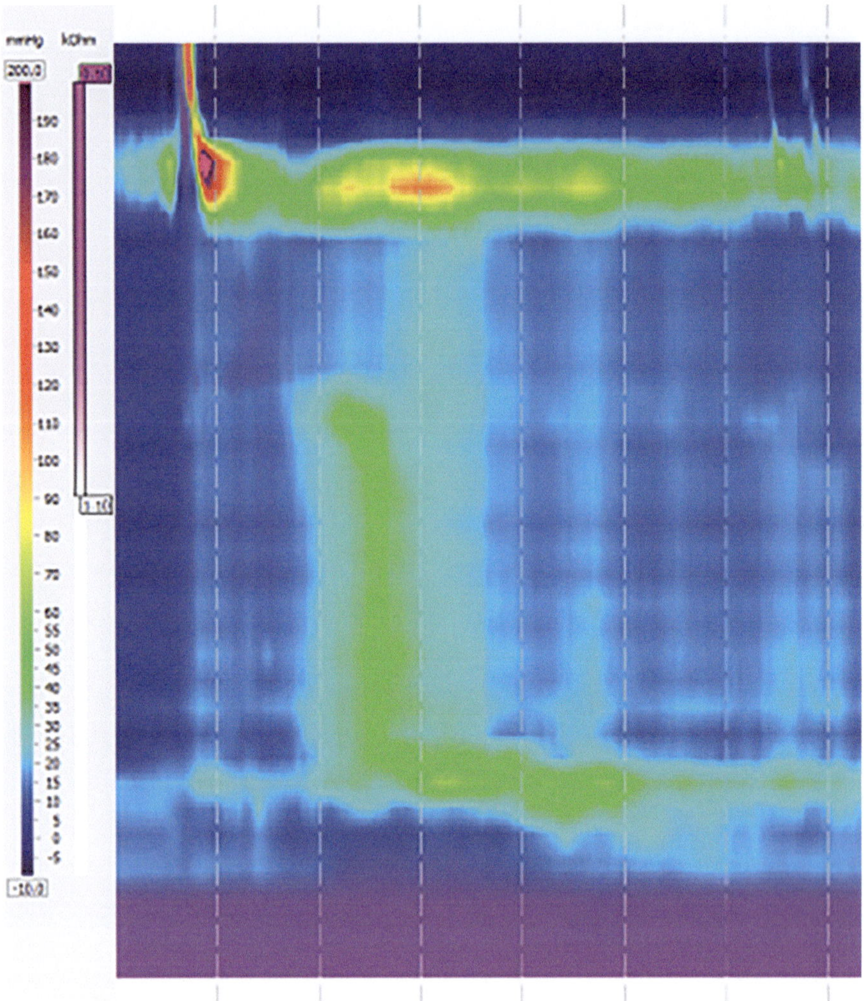

Fig. 9.3 High-resolution manometry showing achalasia, type II

retained fluid, foam, or solid food debris. Patients with achalasia are more likely to have candida esophagitis which can occur secondary to chronic stasis within the esophagus. Additional endoscopic findings include esophageal mucosal changes consistent with chronic stasis (Fig. 9.8).

- EGD helps rule out coexisting or alternative pathology such as stricture, submucosal tumor, esophageal cancer, esophagitis, diverticulum, and hiatal/paraesophageal hernia. These findings impact decisions about further diagnostic testing and treatment.
- Additional studies may be helpful in determining a coexisting and/or alternative diagnoses; however, these studies are not required in every patient. CT chest or PET CT can be helpful to evaluate tumors of the esophagus or GEJ. Endoscopic

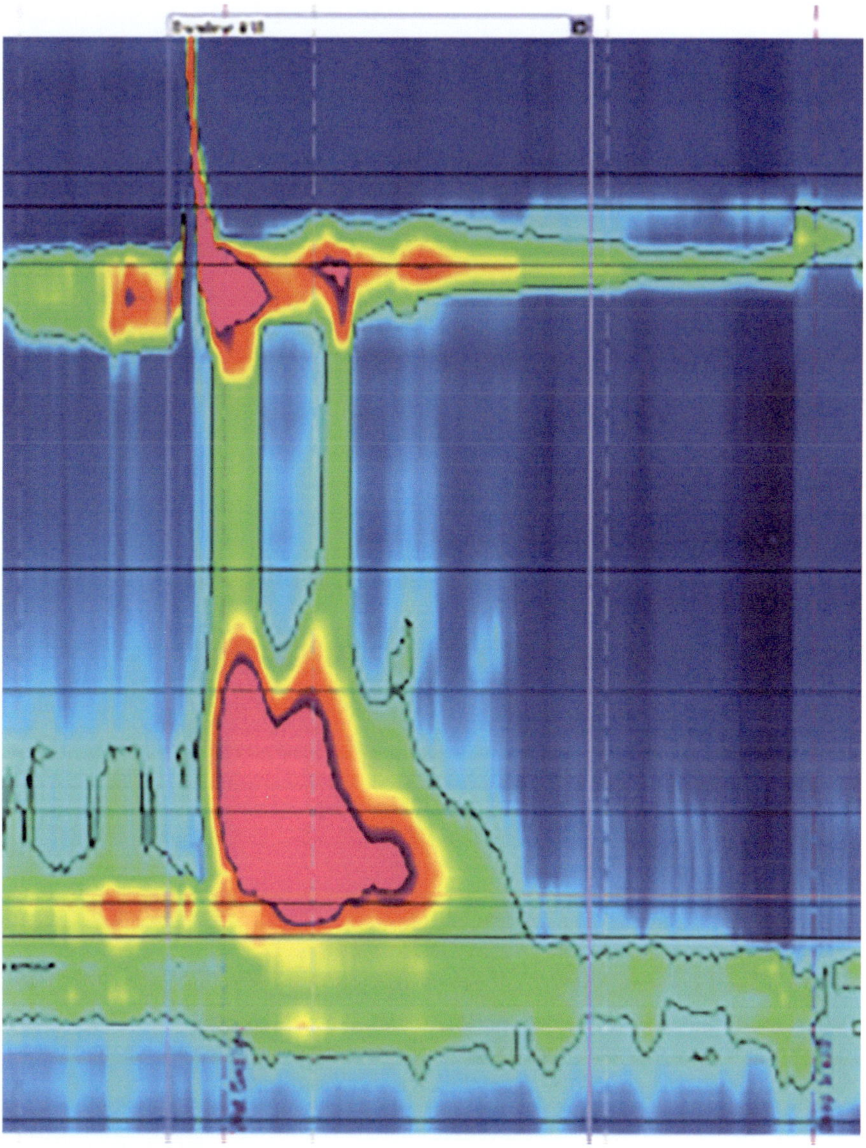

Fig. 9.4 High-resolution manometry showing achalasia, type III

ultrasound (EUS) can also be helpful to evaluate tumors of the esophagus or GEJ. Some achalasia patients may present with aspiration due to regurgitation. At times, there may be uncertainty if coexisting oropharyngeal swallowing dysfunction is contributing to aspiration events. A videofluoroscopic swallowing study (VFSS) can help determine if oropharyngeal dysphagia is contributing to the symptom profile.

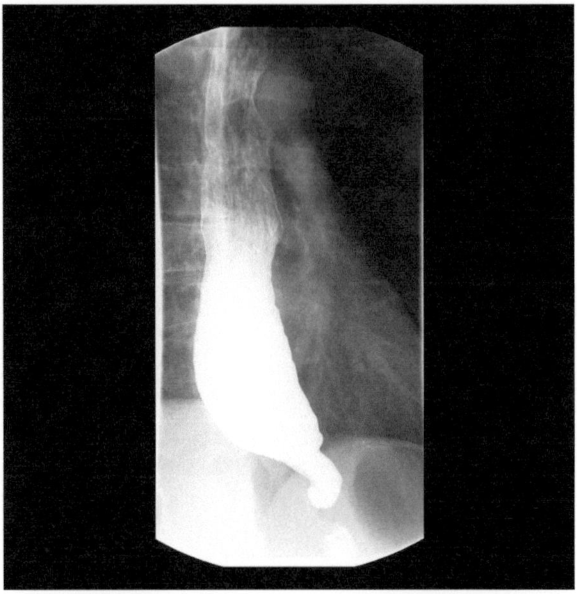

Fig. 9.5 Contrast esophagram in a patient with achalasia

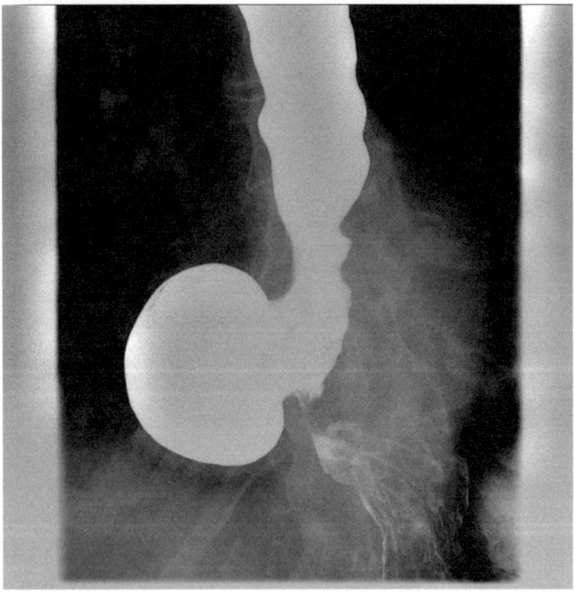

Fig. 9.6 Contrast esophagram in a patient with an epiphrenic diverticulum

Preoperative Preparation

- There is variability regarding preoperative preparation prior to a POEM procedure. Our local process includes preoperative assessment of fitness for surgery

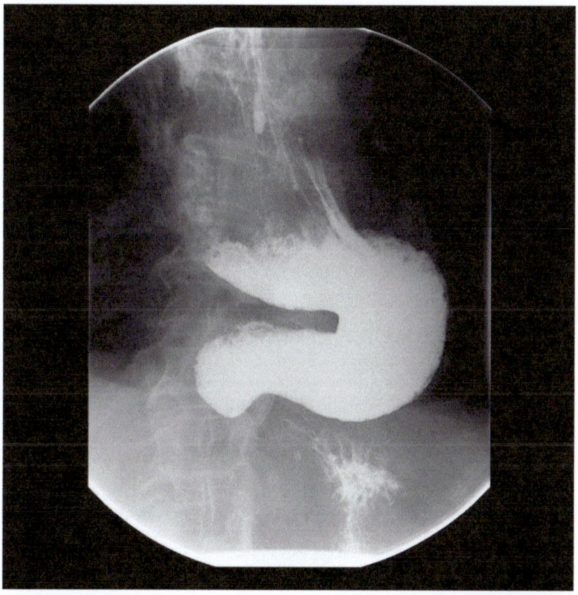

Fig. 9.7 Contrast esophagram in a patient with achalasia and a sigmoid esophagus

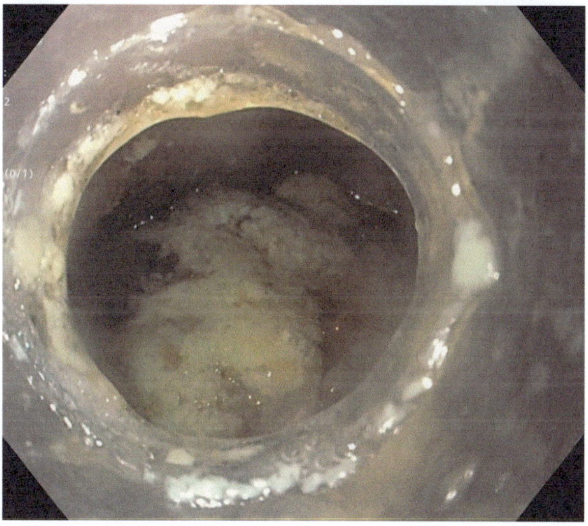

Fig. 9.8 EGD showing retained solid debris in the esophagus

within 1 month prior to the planned procedure, treatment with Nystatin liquid suspension started 3 days prior to the procedure, as well as treatment with fluconazole 200 mg orally times one dose.

- A clear liquid diet is started 48 hours prior to the procedure. Patients with large amounts of solid debris may require longer than 48 hours to achieve adequate clearance of debris.

- Therapeutic anticoagulation, Plavix, and/or high-dose aspirin medications are held in the perioperative period.
- Patients receive cefazolin IV preoperatively according to Surgical Care Improvement Project (SCIP) protocol.
- Patients undergo general endotracheal anesthesia using rapid sequence intubation (RSI), and aspiration prevention protocols are utilized due to the higher risk of aspiration in achalasia patients.
- Performance of the procedure in the operating room versus the GI lab is determined by local of appropriate anesthesia support, specialized equipment, and qualified support staff for utilization of the equipment. We perform the procedure in the operating room.

Technique

Planning

- Equipment includes a standard high-resolution endoscope, endoscope tower, monitor(s), and a CO_2 regulation unit. The scope must be capable of endoscopic irrigation and is fitted with a dissection cap; we prefer a beveled cap.
- An endoscopic injection needle may be used for injection of dyed saline versus a lifting agent; we utilize dyed saline composed of 2 mL of methylene blue in a 1000 mL bag of normal saline. An endoscopic knife with electrosurgical generator is required. We prefer a hybrid knife that combines injection or hydrodissection with electrosurgical energy application.
- A coagrasper hemostatic forceps with active cord is available along with endoscopic closure device(s) including endoscopic clips, over-the-scope clips (OTSC), and/or an endoscopic suturing device.
- A Functional Lumenal Impedance Planimetry (EndoFLIP) device and EndoFLIP catheter are not required to perform the myotome, but are extremely helpful in determining the adequacy of the myotomy.

Endoscopic Access and Anatomical Landmarks

- Patients are placed in the supine position, a bite block is placed with the endotracheal tube placed off to one side. The grounding pad is placed on patient's back.
- An endoscopic assessment is performed and fluid or debris within the esophagus is cleared. For most cases, the overtube is not necessary; however, in an extremely dilated and tortuous esophagus, the overtube can reduce looping.
- Preprocedure EndoFLIP measurements are obtained to establish a baseline. A beveled endoscopic cap is placed. The equipment is checked, ensuring that CO_2

is activated and air is turned off. Endoscopic measurements are taken, with emphasis on determining the distance to the GEJ.

Procedure

- A starting point is identified about 10 cm above GEJ. Some favor a longer myotomy for achalasia type III and/or spastic motility disorders. In these cases, we generally measure the length of the spastic segment based on preoperative high-resolution manometry, and we start 2–3 cm proximal to the top of spastic segment. The optimal myotomy length is still under active investigation, but we continue to utilize the data established for the Heller myotomy of 7 cm on the esophagus and 2–3 cm on the stomach for cases of achalasia type I and II.
- Orientation of the endoscope is determined by allowing fluid to pool posteriorly. There is variability in the preferred orientation of approach. Data currently suggests no significant difference in safety or efficacy of the anterior versus posterior approach. The anterior approach should be offset at the 1–2 o'clock position. The posterior approach should be offset at the 5 o'clock position. It is important to avoid the angle of His and to avoid the lesser curve.

Mucosotomy and Entrance into the Submucosal Space

- The injection needle is used to create a mucosal bleb using dyed saline or a commercial lifting agent (Figs. 9.9 and 9.10). The endoscopic knife is used to create a 1.5–2 cm longitudinal mucosotomy (Figs. 9.11 and 9.12).

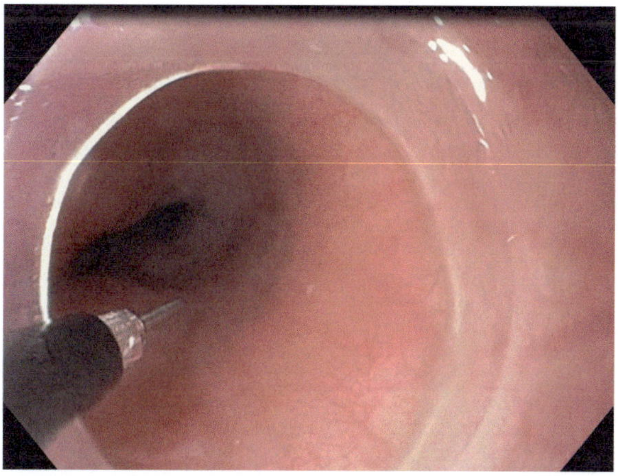

Fig. 9.9 Injection needle prior to mucosal bleb

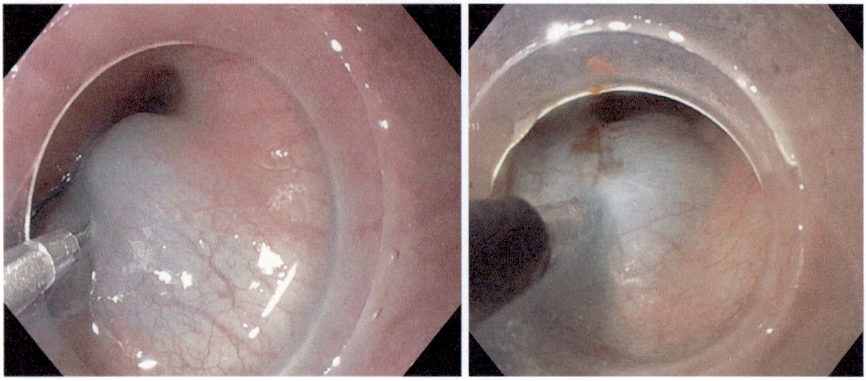

Fig. 9.10 Mucosal bleb

Fig. 9.11 Start of mucosotomy

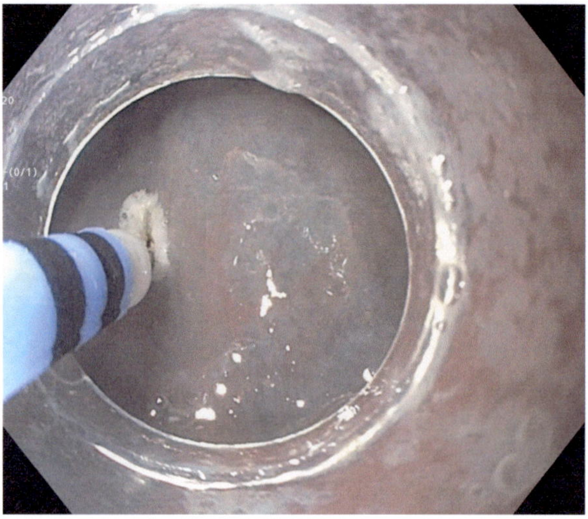

- Additional dyed saline is injected into the submucosal space to lift the mucosa away from the circular muscle fibers. It is usually necessary to lyse some of the submucosal fibers and create space under the mucosa *before* attempting advancement of the endoscope into the submucosal space (Fig. 9.13). The endoscope is then advanced into the submucosal space.

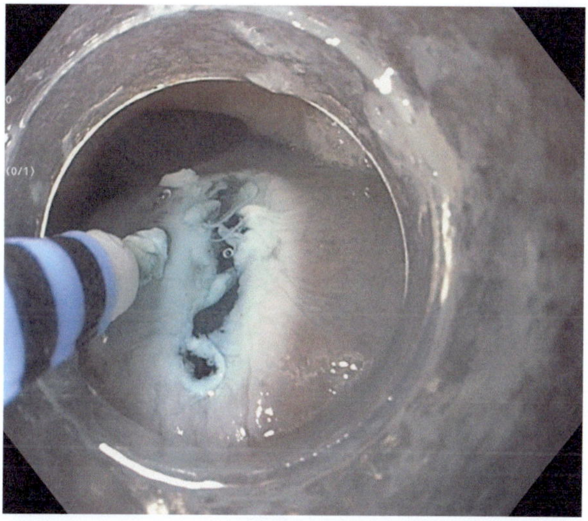

Fig. 9.12 Completed mucosotomy

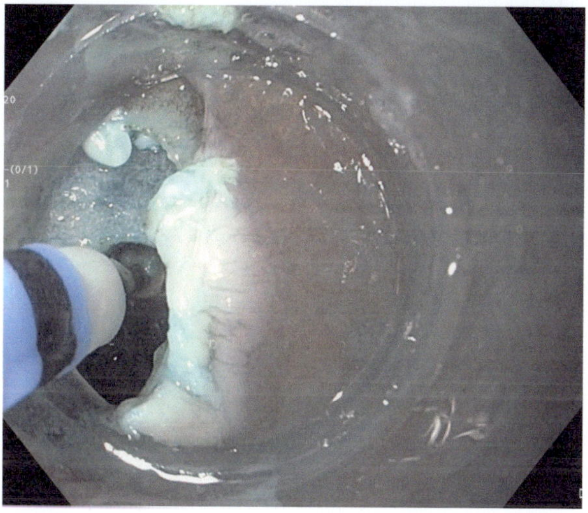

Fig. 9.13 Lysing submucosal fibers prior to entering submucosal space

Creation of Submucosal Tunnel

- Frequent and liberal injection of dyed saline into the submucosal space will aid in lifting the mucosa away from the muscle. The solution will dye the submucosal fibers blue but will not dye the muscle fibers. The endoscopic knife is used to lyse submucosal fibers.
- It is ideal to hug the circular muscle layer and maximize the distance away from the mucosa for the dissection plane (Fig. 9.14). Inadvertent cautery burns to the muscle layer are insignificant since the circular muscle layer will be cut later in the case; however, a thermal injury to the mucosa can create a full thickness

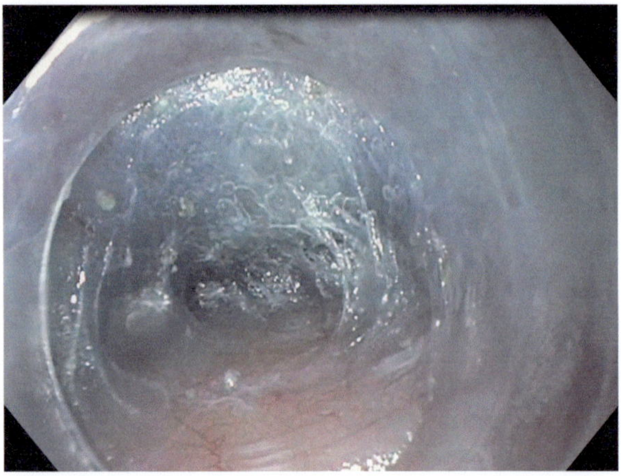

Fig. 9.14 Submucosal tunnel with dissection plane close to the circular muscle fibers

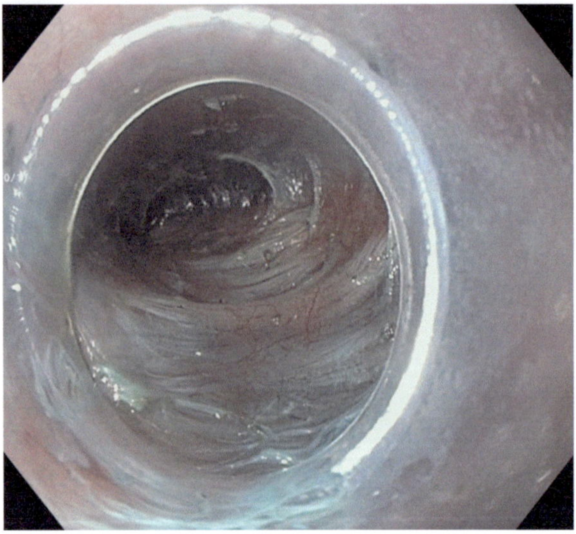

Fig. 9.15 Submucosal tunnel oriented perpendicular to circular muscle fibers

injury. Circular fibers are kept perpendicular to the endoscope which prevents spiraling of the tunnel or migrating of the tunnel to a lateral approach (Fig. 9.15).

- The tunnel width should be one-third to one-half of the circumference of the esophagus. A tunnel that becomes too narrow limits movement of the endoscope. This significantly increases the difficulty of dissection and the management of bleeding. Additionally, a narrow tunnel reduces working space such that inadvertent thermal injury to the mucosa becomes more difficult to avoid (Fig. 9.16).
- The tunnel is extended at least 2 cm onto the stomach. The tunnel endpoint can be determined using a combination of endoscopic measurements, the appearance of the gastric muscle (gastric muscle is paler with palisading vessels), the dual scope technique, and the appearance of tunnel flap and/or dye on retroflexion from within the true gastric lumen (Fig. 9.17).

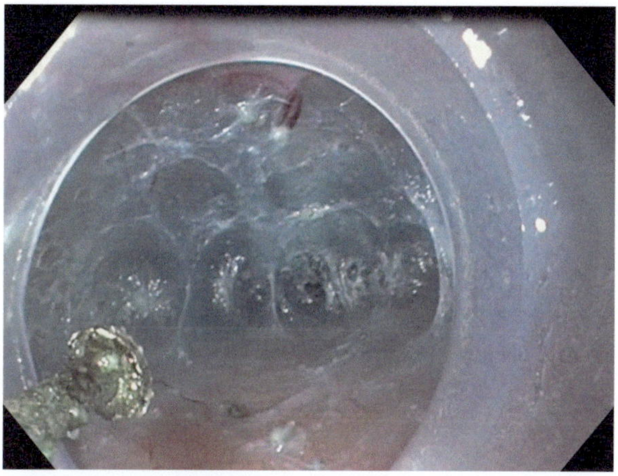

Fig. 9.16 Wide submucosal tunnel

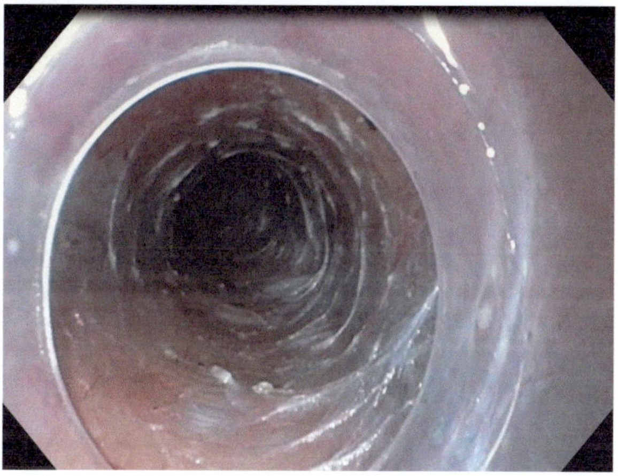

Fig. 9.17 Completed submucosal tunnel

Endoscopic Myotomy

- The myotomy is started 2–3 cm distal to mucosotomy. There is no data to support a proximal-to-distal (antegrade) versus distal-to-proximal (retrograde) approach to the myotomy. We have found that progressing proximal to distal is easier and less time consuming.
- There is variability regarding the desired depth of myotomy (Fig. 9.18). Some attempt to perform a circular muscle fiber myotomy, while others perform a full-thickness myotomy. Initial data suggest a shorter procedure time with full-thickness myotomy but otherwise equivalent safety and efficacy (Fig. 9.19). We generally attempt to perform a circular muscle fiber myotomy; however, at the GEJ, we create a full-thickness myotomy (Fig. 9.20). The myotomy should extend at least 2 cm onto the stomach.

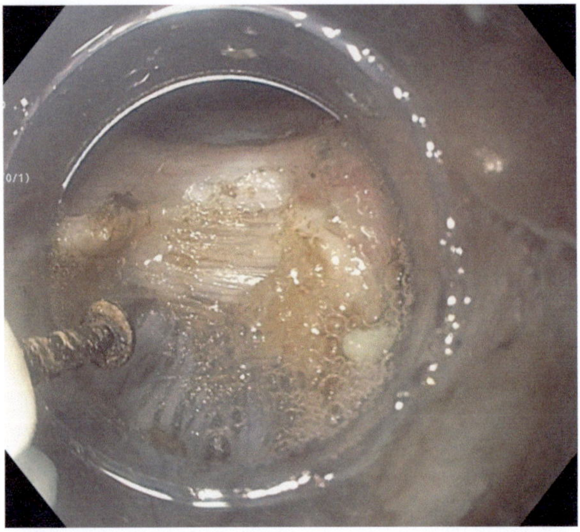

Fig. 9.18 Visualization of circular and longitudinal muscle fibers

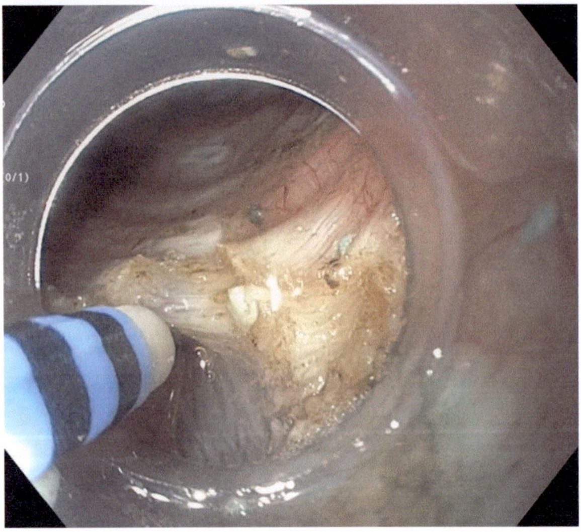

Fig. 9.19 Myotomy of circular muscle fibers

- The extent of the myotomy can be assessed with endoscopic measurements, the dual scope technique, the appearance of tunnel flap and/or dye on retroflexion from within the true gastric lumen, or by using the EndoFLIP catheter.

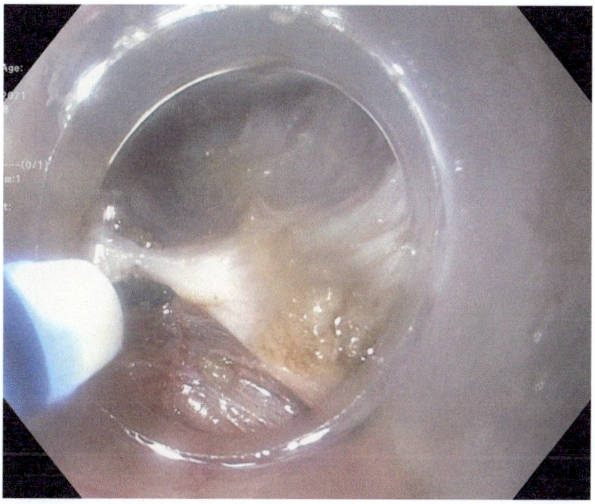

Fig. 9.20 Full-thickness myotomy

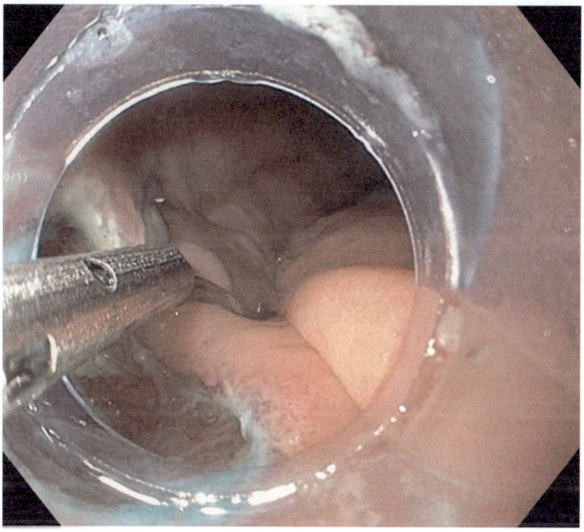

Fig. 9.21 Orientation of first clip distal to the myotomy

Closure of the Mucosotomy

- Prior to closure, the mucosa along the tunnel should be assessed for perforations and thermal injuries. Perforations or thermal injuries can be managed with endoscopic clips from within the true esophageal lumen.
- Closure of the mucosotomy can be performed with a variety of methods. When using endoscopic clips, it is often easiest to apply the first clip slightly distal to the mucosotomy (Figs. 9.21 and 9.22). This helps to elevate and evert the edges of the mucosotomy to facilitate subsequent clip placement (Fig. 9.23).
- Other methods may involve an endoscopic suturing device such as the Apollo Overstitch or the Apollo X-tack or over-the-scope clips (OTSC).

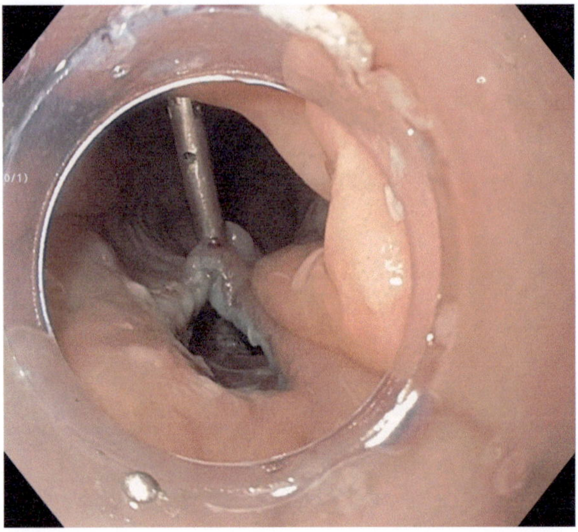

Fig. 9.22 View after first clip has been placed

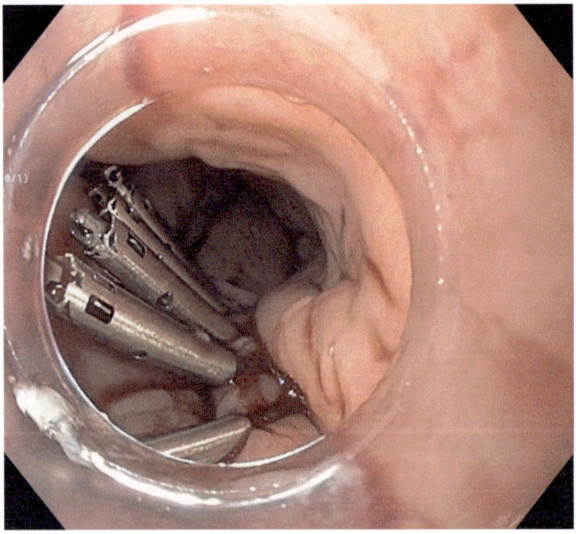

Fig. 9.23 Clip closure of mucosotomy

Postoperative Care

- The procedure is performed as outpatient or as an overnight stay. Factors such as comorbid medical conditions and/or operative findings may require a longer inpatient stay.
- Routine esophagram is not necessary in every patient.
- We start a clear liquid diet when the patient is awake and advance to a Nissen diet as tolerated. Patients remain on a Nissen diet until the 2-week follow-up. If they are doing well, the diet is then advanced.
- We routinely start all patients on a once daily PPI following surgery and recommend continuing this indefinitely which mirrors our management of patients who undergo Heller myotomy. Alternatively, if patients desire to avoid acid suppression medications, then objective testing should be performed to guide the conversation about use of long-term acid suppression. No guidelines exist regarding routine surveillance endoscopy or pH testing. We generally recommend surveillance endoscopy every 3–5 years. Further testing is generally reserved for patients who develop new or recurrent symptoms or who wish to avoid acid suppression medications.
- Most patients notice an immediate improvement in their achalasia symptoms; however, symptom improvement generally continues for several weeks as recovery from surgery progresses. The most common patient concerns include sore throat, retrosternal chest discomfort, and heartburn.

Outcomes

- The clinical efficacy of POEM for achalasia is >90% out to 3-year follow-up [10]. Overall, these rates are uniformly higher than for Heller myotomy with partial fundoplication, but this does not reach statistical significance. The efficacy wanes to 82% at longer-term follow-up >5 years [10]. Efficacy is similar for both type I and type II achalasia.
- POEM and Heller myotomy with partial fundoplication are considered equivalent in efficacy for types I and II achalasia. The efficacy of POEM for type III achalasia is modestly higher than the efficacy of Heller myotomy with partial fundoplication, and this difference is statistically significant Therefore, most regard POEM as the preferred approach for patients with type III achalasia.
- POEM is both safe and effective in the setting of prior treatment failures (prior Heller myotomy or prior POEM). Comparative data is lacking, but most would agree that reoperation with the endoscopic approach offers a safer approach than reoperation using the laparoscopic approach, especially if an anterior myotomy already exists.
- Gastroesophageal reflux disease (GERD) is a side effect following myotomy. Rates of reflux are reported as subjective (symptom scoring) or objective (pH

testing or visualization of esophagitis on endoscopic evaluation). Subjective rates of GERD after POEM range from 9% to 43% [11, 12]. Objective rates of GERD after POEM range from 13% to 68% [11, 12]. Subjective and objective rates of GERD after POEM are generally higher than after Heller myotomy with partial fundoplication. Some evidence suggests that GERD rates (subjective and objective) decrease in the first year after POEM [11]. Additionally, there is evidence to suggest that GERD rates increase in the years after Heller myotomy with fundoplication [11].

- Patients with achalasia are thought to have a degree of visceral desensitization. Alarmingly, approximately half of patients with objective evidence of GERD report no symptoms of GERD.
- Studies evaluating the impact of tunnel orientation, length of myotomy, depth of myotomy, and EndoFLIP measurements on postoperative GERD have not yielded consistent results. There is some initial data suggesting that gastric sling fiber preservation may reduce the rate GERD [11]. Obesity increases the risk for development of GERD after POEM by five-fold. Patients should be preoperatively counseled regarding this risk [10].

Pearls	Pitfalls
Vessels bridging the submucosal space	Proactively cauterize these with either the endoscopic knife or the coagraspers Stay near muscle when doing this so that if the vessel retracts toward the mucosa after being cut, there may still be an end that can be grasped
Bleeding in the tunnel	Bleeding can occur from a partial defect in a vessel or from a transected end of a vessel. Bleeding in the tunnel does not generally involve massive blood loss; rather, bleeding in a small space can significantly impair visualization such that operative progress cannot continue. If the bleeding is easily visualized, then cautery using the endoscopic knife can be applied or a coagrasper can be utilized to grab and cauterize Bleeders along the mucosal side of the dissection must be addressed with care to avoid thermal injuries to the mucosa. Gentle pressure with the endoscopic cap and/or the blunt tip of an endoscopic knife can be used to tamponade bleeding without the use of energy. Grasping and gently pulling away from the mucosa can be a useful technique If blood is welling up too quickly to visualize the bleeding or blood is welling up such that the cautery is not effective, then we use the following technique (Fig. 9.24). Center the cap over the area of bleeding and apply gentler pressure. Flood the distal tunnel using the water pump until the underwater view is clear. Halt the water pump and watch for a puff of blood to locate the bleeding vessel (Figs. 9.25 and 9.26). Use the coagrasper to grasp the bleeding area or use the blunt end of the endoscopic knife to tamponade the exact site of bleeding. Suction out the fluid and insufflate some CO_2 to dry the area. Apply gentle cautery (Fig. 9.27)

(continued)

Pearls	Pitfalls
Mucosal defects	Identifying mucosal defects is important Clips or endoscopic suturing devices can be used to close the defect from within the true esophageal lumen Defects at the GEJ can be a significant challenge as the approach can be difficult Defects that cannot be closed may be managed with a stent
Tight tunnel at the GEJ that does not allow passage of the endoscope	Back up and ensure that the tunnel is sufficiently wide as it approaches the GEJ Consider performing the myotomy to open this area up and facilitate further submucosal dissection beyond the GEJ
Crepitus	This represents tracking of CO_2 throughout the mediastinum This is generally self-limited, but mandates inpatient observation until resolved
Capnoperitoneum	We utilize a Veress needle at the end of the case if this occurs An area in the left upper quadrant is prepped and draped in a sterile fashion. A 3-mm skin nick is created. The Veress needle is inserted to allow for decompression of the peritoneal cavity
Capnothorax	Patients may develop capnothorax which is seldom symptomatic If there are no respiratory symptoms, then expectant management without intervention is sufficient as the CO_2 will dissipate If respiratory symptoms are present, then pigtail catheter drainage can be performed
Post-procedure bleeding into the tunnel	Bleeding into the tunnel after the procedure can result in a large submucosal hematoma which can partially obstruct the distal esophageal lumen and result in persistent dysphagia as well as pain. If the blood expresses through the mucosotomy, then hematemesis can result If the patient can tolerate liquids but has persistent symptoms, then watchful waiting can be pursued and the hematoma will generally resolve Several options have been described for patients who are unable to tolerate oral intake such a utilizing TPN or a surgical feeding tube or endoscopic evacuation of the hematoma and management of the bleeding if it can be located Bleeding with hematemesis generally requires endoscopic evaluation, evacuation of hematoma, and management of bleeding
Esophageal leak	This is an uncommon but feared complication of POEM Management of leaks is often determined by the symptomatic presentation. Clips or stents may be adequate for an early leak with minimal contamination. In more severe presentations, drainage of the chest may be necessary Attention to alternative routes of nutrition is necessary

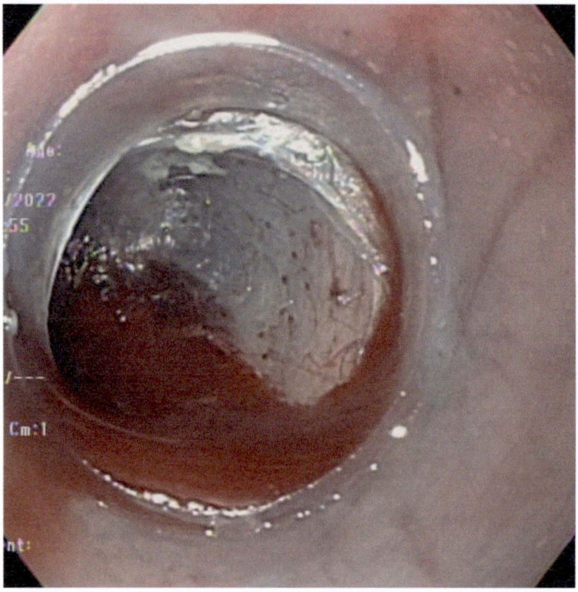

Fig. 9.24 Bleeding in the submucosal tunnel

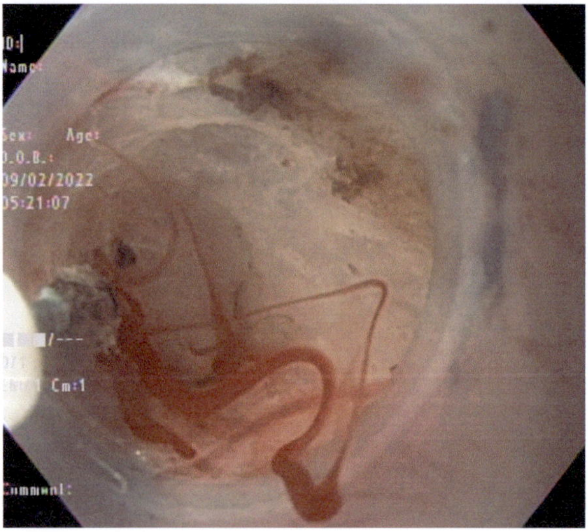

Fig. 9.25 Bleeding vessel submerged

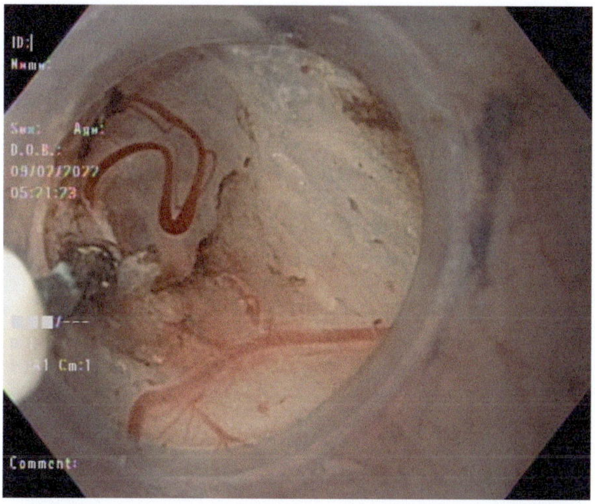

Fig. 9.26 Cauterization of bleeding vessel

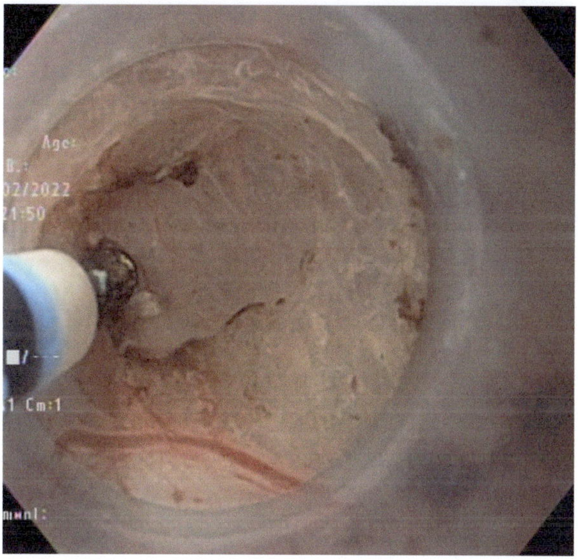

Fig. 9.27 Hemostasis

References

1. Crema E, Ferreira DA, Silva AA, Ferreira-Santos R. Análise comparativa de três tipos de válvulas anti-refluxo associada à cirurgia de Heller: estudo experimental em cães. Rev Col Bras Cir. 2002;29:249–55.
2. Ortega JA, Madureri V, Perez L. Endoscopic myotomy in the treatment of achalasia. Gastrointest Endosc. 1980;26(1):8–10.
3. Sumiyama K, Gostout CJ, Rajan E, Bakken TA, Knipschield MA. Transesophageal mediastinoscopy by submucosal endoscopy with mucosal flap safety valve technique. Gastrointest Endosc. 2007;65(4):679–83. Available from: https://pubmed.ncbi.nlm.nih.gov/17383463/

4. Pasricha PJ, Hawarl R, Ahmed I, Chen J, Cotton PB, Hawes RH, et al. Submucosal endoscopic esophageal myotomy: a novel experimental approach for the treatment of achalasia. Endoscopy. 2007;39(9):761–4. Available from: https://pubmed.ncbi.nlm.nih.gov/17703382/
5. Inoue H, Minami H, Kobayashi Y, Sato Y, Kaga M, Suzuki M, et al. Peroral endoscopic myotomy (POEM) for esophageal achalasia. Endoscopy. 2010;42(4):265–71. Available from: https://pubmed.ncbi.nlm.nih.gov/20354937/
6. Kohn GP, Dirks RC, Ansari MT, Clay J, Dunst CM, Lundell L, et al. SAGES guidelines for the use of peroral endoscopic myotomy (POEM) for the treatment of achalasia. Surg Endosc. 2021;35(5):1931–48. Available from: https://research.monash.edu/en/publications/sages-guidelines-for-the-use-of-peroral-endoscopic-myotomy-poem-f
7. Vaezi MF, Pandolfino JE, Yadlapati RH, Greer KB, Kavitt RT. ACG clinical guidelines: diagnosis and management of Achalasia. Am J Gastroenterol. 2020;115(9):1393–411. Available from: https://pubmed.ncbi.nlm.nih.gov/32773454/
8. Khashab MA, Vela MF, Thosani N, Agrawal D, Buxbaum JL, Abbas Fehmi SM, et al. ASGE guideline on the management of achalasia. Gastrointest Endosc. 2020;91(2):213–227.e6. Available from: https://pubmed.ncbi.nlm.nih.gov/31839408/
9. Yadlapati R, Kahrilas PJ, Fox MR, Bredenoord AJ, Prakash Gyawali C, Roman S, Babaei A, Mittal RK, Rommel N, Savarino E, Sifrim D. Esophageal motility disorders on high-resolution manometry: Chicago classification version 4.0©. Neurogastroenterol Motil. 2021;33(1):e14058.
10. Zhang H, Zeng X, Huang S, Shi L, Xia H, Jiang J, et al. Mid-term and long-term outcomes of peroral endoscopic myotomy for the treatment of achalasia: a systematic review and meta-analysis. Dig Dis Sci. 2023;68(4):1386–96. Available from: https://pubmed.ncbi.nlm.nih.gov/36260203/
11. Rassoul Abu-Nuwar M, Eriksson SE, Sarici IS, Zheng P, Hoppo T, Jobe BA, et al. GERD after peroral endoscopic myotomy: assessment of incidence and predisposing factors. J Am Coll Surg. 2023;236(1):58–70. Available from: https://pubmed.ncbi.nlm.nih.gov/36519909/
12. Sharma P, Stavropoulos SN. Is peroral endoscopic myotomy the new gold standard for achalasia therapy? Dig Endosc. 2023;35(2):173–83. Available from: https://pubmed.ncbi.nlm.nih.gov/36385512/

Chapter 10
Peroral Endoscopic Myotomy for Zenker's Diverticulum (ZPOEM)

Lucas Fair and Marc A. Ward

Background

- Zenker's diverticulum (ZD) is an uncommon disorder characterized by a saclike outpouching of the mucosal and submucosal layers that occur at Killian's triangle [1]. The etiology of ZD is not completely understood. It is believed that repeated, high pharyngeal pressure during swallowing eventually causes herniation of the posterior pharyngeal wall between the inferior pharyngeal constrictor and the cricopharyngeus. The prevalence of ZD ranges from 0.01% to 0.11% of the population, most commonly affecting elderly males [2].
- Patients with small diverticula can be asymptomatic. Early in the disease course, patients may note transient dysphagia. As diverticula get larger, they can retain foreign materials such as food, sputum, and medications. Patients with enlarging diverticula can experience dysphagia, halitosis, choking, and recurrent aspiration [3]. Weight loss and malnutrition can occur in patients with long-term dysphagia.

L. Fair
Department of Minimally Invasive Surgery, Baylor University Medical Center, Dallas, TX, USA

Center for Advanced Surgery, Baylor Scott and White Health, Dallas, TX, USA

Research Institute, Dallas, TX, USA
e-mail: Lucas.Fair@bswhealth.org

M. A. Ward (✉)
Department of Minimally Invasive Surgery, Baylor University Medical Center, Dallas, TX, USA

Center for Advanced Surgery, Baylor Scott and White Health, Dallas, TX, USA

Texas A&M College of Medicine, Bryan, TX, USA
e-mail: marc.ward@BSWHealth.org

M. Ujiki, Z. M. Callahan (eds.), *Third Space Endoscopy*,
https://doi.org/10.1007/978-3-031-84509-3_10

- Patients with a ZD may require surgical treatment, which can be performed via an open surgical or endoscopic approach. Open surgical techniques have had high success rates, but have the potential for serious surgical morbidity [4]. Conventional endoscopic techniques are less invasive than open surgery with improved morbidity rates. However, endoscopic approaches have also been associated with high recurrence rates that have been reported between 7% and 24% [5].
- A new technique called peroral endoscopic myotomy (POEM) has recently been developed to treat various gastrointestinal pathologies. POEM relies on creating a submucosal tunnel that enables access to the muscularis propria so that a complete myotomy can be performed endoscopically. This tunnel-assisted technique has now been incorporated into the treatment armamentarium for ZD to offer an improved minimally invasive approach. A benefit of this technique is that it allows for complete exposure and dissection of the cricopharyngeal muscle fibers in the septum between the esophagus and diverticulum. This makes a more liberal myotomy possible, which can reduce recurrence rates secondary to an incomplete septotomy. This technique is colloquially referred to as ZPOEM, and it has emerged as a promising new treatment for ZD.
- The purpose of this chapter is to evaluate the indications, technical steps, pearls and pitfalls, and outcomes when using this technique for the treatment of ZD.

Indications

- Patients with small, asymptomatic ZD less than 1 centimeter do not require treatment and can be managed conservatively until symptoms occur. For patients with symptomatic or larger ZD ($\geq$1 centimeter), ZPOEM can be considered for definitive management.
- Since the presence of ZD is a risk for aspiration, patients are induced under general anesthesia with rapid sequence intubation, and thus, the inability to tolerate general anesthesia is a contraindication to ZPOEM.
- ZPOEM may be advantageous for high-risk elderly patients and those with histories of previous neck operations due to the minimally invasive nature of the procedure [6]. ZPOEM may offer a benefit in patients with symptomatic, small diverticula in comparison to other treatment modalities. It is well known that small (<1 cm) pouches have worse outcomes after a traditional endoscopic approach [7]. This is primarily due to the short common wall between the esophagus and pouch, which makes the septum difficult to divide completely using traditional endoscopic methods.
- ZPOEM may offer an advantage over other endoscopic modalities because it can achieve a complete myotomy extending onto the posterior esophageal muscle over several centimeters due to the secure closure of the mucosotomy.

Patient Evaluation

Initial Evaluation

- Validated symptom assessments should be obtained from all patients to quantify symptom severity upon initial presentation. There are several symptom assessment tools available, and the one used is left to the discretion of the surgeon or endoscopist [8, 9]. This should be obtained to effectively determine whether there is symptomatic improvement after the procedure.

Diagnostic Studies

- The presence of a ZD is typically established by upper endoscopy and/or barium esophagram (Fig. 10.1). An alternative imaging method to diagnose ZD is a transcutaneous ultrasound, which can be used in patients who have difficulty swallowing barium or cannot undergo upper endoscopy [10].

Preoperative Preparation

- Patients are started on a liquid diet for 2–5 days before the procedure to ensure a clear endoscopic view and avoid aspiration of diverticulum contents during induction of anesthesia.

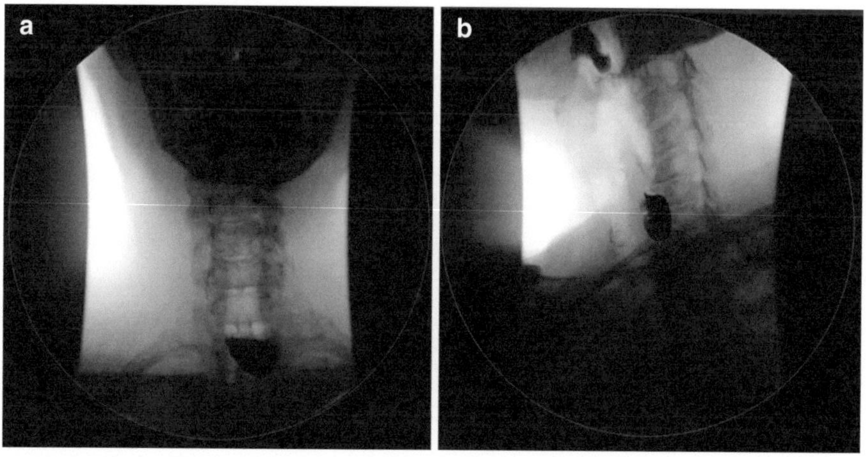

Fig. 10.1 Barium swallow demonstrating contrast within a Zenker's diverticulum (**a**, **b**)

- Nystatin 200,000 IU solution four times per day is given for 5 days before the surgery. If feasible, anticoagulant or antiplatelet medications should be held perioperatively. Prophylactic intravenous antibiotics are usually not necessary, but can be given if desired. Intravenous dexamethasone (6–8 mg) can be given at the time of surgery to reduce swelling during the procedure.
- Deep vein thrombosis (DVT) prophylaxis is usually not necessary for this procedure unless the patient is at high risk for a thrombotic event with a low risk for bleeding.

Technique

Planning

- A high-definition flexible endoscope, loaded with an endoscopic cap, is used for the entirety of the procedure. Carbon dioxide can be used for insufflation at a low flow rate and not air as this can lead to subcutaneous emphysema or a pneumothorax [11].
- A mixture of saline stained with either methylene blue or indigo carmine can be used for the submucosal injection and development of the submucosal tunnel. Multiple electrosurgical devices can be used for the submucosal tunnel formation and myotomy, which most commonly includes knife devices. Standard endoscopic clips are used to close the initial mucosal incision.

Endoscopic Access and Anatomical Landmarks

- Once patients are in the operating room, they are placed in the supine position and induced under general anesthesia with rapid sequence intubation due to the high aspiration risk. Left lateral decubitus is an alternative patient position that can be used [11].
- First, a diagnostic upper endoscopy is performed with a focus on the visualization of the diverticulum. If there is a retained food bolus, it should be carefully removed to prevent an aspiration event.

Procedure

- The submucosa proximal to the ZD septum is injected with a mixture of saline and methylene blue to create a submucosal bleb (Fig. 10.2a). This same mixture is used throughout the case to infiltrate the submucosal space and to assist in hydrodissection.
- A mucosal incision of 1–2 cm length is then created to enter and create a submucosal tunnel entry point (Fig. 10.2b). Next, the endoscope enters the submucosal space with the aid of the endoscopic cap.
- The submucosal fibers are dissected, and the submucosal tunnel is created using electrocautery and injection of methylene blue until the thick diverticular septum is identified (Fig. 10.2c).
- The tunnel is continued on both the diverticular side and esophageal side until the bottom of the diverticulum is reached and the septum of the cricopharyngeus is entirely exposed.
- Once the cricopharyngeal is entirely exposed, the septotomy is performed. Under direct endoscopic view, the muscle fibers of the septum are completely divided using the ERBEJET® (Erbe USA, Incorporated, 2225 Northwest Parkway,

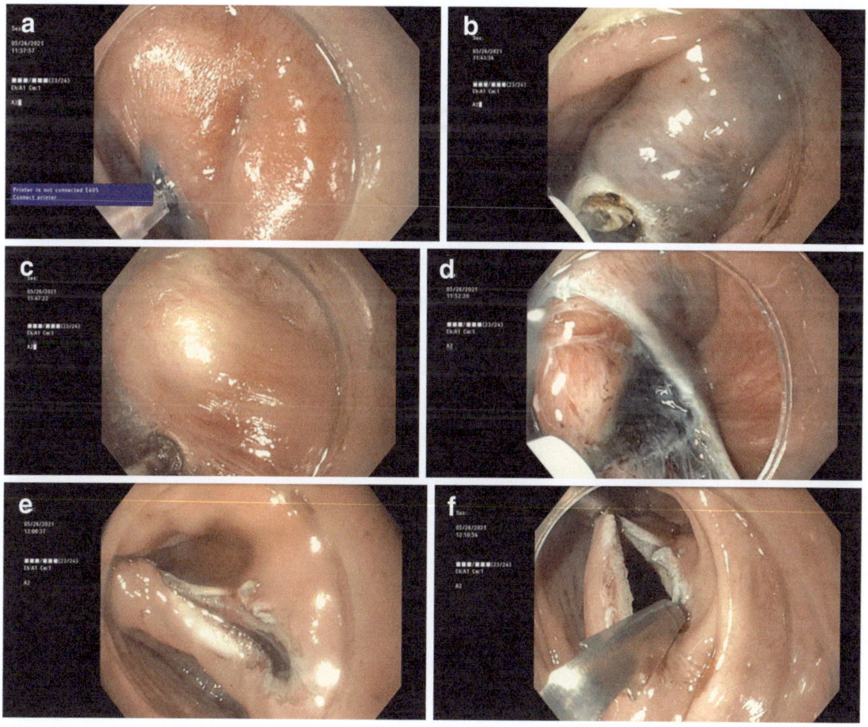

Fig. 10.2 Visualization throughout the ZPOEM procedure: submucosal wheel (**a**), mucosotomy (**b**), submucosal tunnel (**c**), myotomy (**d**), and closure (**e, f**)

Marietta, Georgia 30,067, USA) with a cut/coagulation hybrid function (Fig. 10.2d). The scope is withdrawn from the submucosa and returned into the esophageal lumen.

- Once hemostasis is confirmed with no incidental mucosal entries noted, the mucosal defect is closed using endoscopic clips. The initial clip is placed at the most distal part of the incision with subsequent clips placed in a distal to proximal direction until the mucosal incision is completely closed (Fig. 10.2e–f).
- After the mucosal incision is closed, the endoscope is withdrawn, and the patient is awakened from anesthesia and taken to post anesthesia recovery unit.

Postoperative Care

- Patients are admitted overnight for observation, and antiemetics are given prophylactically. We do not routinely continue antibiotics after surgery.
- The patient is kept *nil* per os, and an esophagram is obtained on postoperative day 1 to exclude an esophageal leak (Fig. 10.3). If no leak is identified, the patient is started on a liquid diet and subsequently discharged if stable.
- Patients are advised to stay on a liquid diet for 1 week postoperatively and then can advance to a regular diet as tolerated. This is done to prevent dislodgement of the endoscopic clips.
- Patients follow up in 2–4 weeks after their surgery via an in-person clinic visit or telehealth. Patients are assessed for any delayed complications and clinical

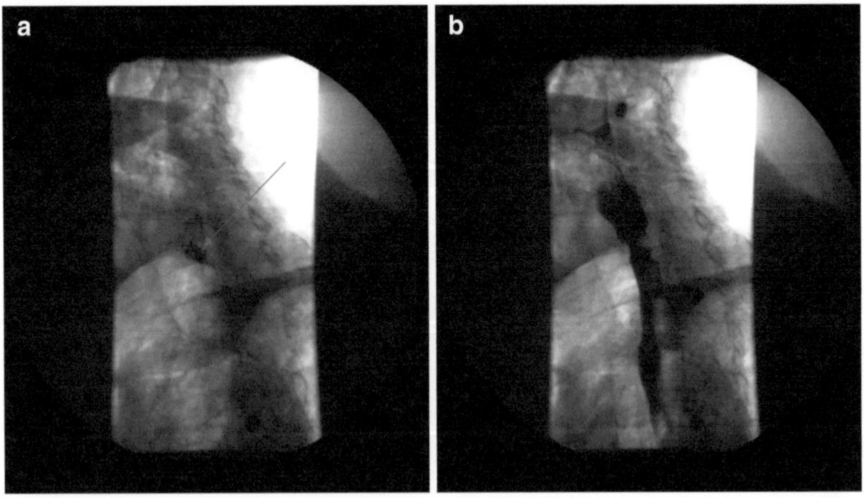

Fig. 10.3 Postoperative barium esophagram obtained after ZPOEM before (**a**) and after barium swallow (**b**) demonstrating no evidence of a leak with an arrow identifying the endoscopic clips used to close the mucosal incision in the cricopharyngeal region (**a**)

response to ZPOEM during subsequent visits. If symptoms return, a repeat barium esophagram should be obtained if there are concerns for a recurrent ZD.

Outcomes

- ZPOEM is a technically feasible and highly efficacious procedure in the short-term management of ZD. According to a 2022 systematic review and meta-analysis summary of 11 studies of ZPOEM, clinical success was achieved in 89.5–100% of patients. Clinical success was defined as a complete or near-complete resolution of symptoms based on various symptom scoring systems, without the need for additional intervention at follow-up. The technical success of the procedure, defined as the completion of all procedural steps, was 96.3%. Reported clinical recurrence rates were reported from 0 to 14.7% [12]. Other recent reviews have documented similar technical and clinical success rates of ZPOEM [13].
- ZPOEM appears to be a relatively safe procedure with an adverse event rate reported from 0% to 16.8%. The most frequent adverse events reported are bleeding, perforations, and gas-related complications. The majority of adverse events patients undergoing ZPOEM have been managed expectantly, medically, or endoscopically [12].
- Ghamdi et al. conducted a multicenter retrospective review evaluating outcomes between different endoscopic approaches. Rigid endoscopy was associated with the highest rate of complications, and flexible endoscopic septotomy (FES) was associated with the lowest rate of complications (30.0% vs. 2.3%, $p < 0.05$). ZPOEM was in between these two approaches, with adverse events occurring at a rate of 16.8%. ZPOEM had a higher rate of clinical success (92.7%) than rigid septotomy (89.2%) and flexible septotomy (86.7%), albeit this was not statistically significant ($p = 0.26$) [14].
- The aforementioned systematic review and analysis by Zhang and colleagues also compared outcomes between ZPOEM and FES. ZPOEM demonstrated a significantly higher clinical success rate (93.0% vs. 87.9%) and potentially had lower rates of clinical recurrence and incidence of adverse events when compared to FES [12].
- Further comparative studies with long-term follow-up are still needed to validate the findings of the studies available in the literature. However, current evidence suggests that ZPOEM is an excellent option for patients suffering from ZD.

Pearls	Pitfalls
Mucosal incision	Be sure to clearly identify the diverticular and esophageal lumens prior to the incision The incision can favor the diverticular side to make closure of the tunnel entry easier at the end of the case Use a mixture of saline and methylene blue without epinephrine Avoid epinephrine as there have been cases of cardiovascular complications and mucosal ischemia reported [12]
Myotomy	Carry the myotomy onto the esophageal muscle for a minimum of 2 cm to ensure complete division of the cricopharyngeus A liberal myotomy can be performed as the tunnel technique affords secure closure independent of the length and depth of the myotomy
Submucosal tunnel	Ensure that the endoscope is properly oriented as it is advanced through the tunnel to preserve the integrity of the mucosal layer Remember, the mucosal layer becomes the only remaining barrier between the mediastinum and the esophageal lumen after myotomy is performed Frequent, repeated injections should be performed to help avoid a mucosal injury Excessive suctioning should be avoided as this can tear blood vessels or cause mucosal lacerations Large blood vessels should be cauterized to maintain hemostasis and a clear operative field Hemorrhage can be controlled temporarily by tamponading the site with the endoscope Bleeding vessels should be precisely cauterized using coagulation forceps for definitive management Be cautious when using cautery to avoid a thermal injury to the mucosa
Closure	Place the initial endoscopic clip at the most distal part of the incision to facilitate improved approximation of the incision borders Correct deployment of the first clip is important because it makes the placement of subsequent clips much easier Most importantly, inadequate closure can lead to adverse events such as leaks If the first clip creates an asymmetric fold that would make closure difficult or unsafe, consider removing it and redeploying the clip correctly Most mucosal incisions can be closed with three to six clips

References

1. Anagiotos A, Preuss SF, Koebke J. Morphometric and anthropometric analysis of Killian's triangle. Laryngoscope. 2010;120(6):1082–8. Available from: https://pubmed.ncbi.nlm.nih.gov/20513021/
2. Nesheiwat Z, Antunes C. Zenker diverticulum. StatPearls; 2023. Available from: https://www.ncbi.nlm.nih.gov/books/NBK499996/
3. Elkholy S, El-Sherbiny M, Delano-Alonso R, et al. Peroral endoscopic myotomy as treatment for Zenker's diverticulum (Z-POEM): a multi-center international study. Esophagus. 2021;18(3):693–9. Available from: https://pubmed.ncbi.nlm.nih.gov/33387150/
4. Yuan Y, Zhao YF, Hu Y, Chen LQ. Surgical treatment of Zenker's diverticulum. Dig Surg. 2013;30(3):207–18. Available from: https://doi.org/10.1159/000351433

5. Cerchione R, Parise P, Olivari G, Cossu A, Barbieri L, Palucci M, et al. Endoscopic management of Zenker's diverticulum: stapling vs. Z-POEM. Shanghai Chest. 2020;4. Available from: https://shc.amegroups.org/article/view/5811/html
6. Hoffmann M, Fazel A, Mews KG, Ambrosch P. 32 years of experience with CO2 -LASER-assisted treatment for Zenker's diverticulum – an update of 227 patients treated in Kiel. Clin Otolaryngol. 2017;42(3):592–6. Available from: https://pubmed.ncbi.nlm.nih.gov/27762065/
7. Bonavina L, Bona D, Abraham M, Saino G, Abate E. Long-term results of endosurgical and open surgical approach for Zenker diverticulum. World J Gastroenterol. 2007;13(18):2586.
8. Crary MA, Carnaby Mann GD, Groher ME. Initial psychometric assessment of a functional oral intake scale for dysphagia in stroke patients. Arch Phys Med Rehabil. 2005;86(8):1516–20. Available from: https://pubmed.ncbi.nlm.nih.gov/16084801/
9. Dakkak M, Bennett JR. A new dysphagia score with objective validation. J Clin Gastroenterol. 1992;14(2):99–100. Available from: https://pubmed.ncbi.nlm.nih.gov/1556441/
10. Jiang L, Hu B, Wang Z, Zhao B. Sonographic diagnosis features of Zenker diverticulum. Eur J Radiol. 2011;80(2) Available from: https://pubmed.ncbi.nlm.nih.gov/20576383/
11. Podgaetz E, Konda V. Experience and technique for Zenker's diverticulum per Oral endoscopic Myotomy: Z-POEM. Thorac Cardiovasc Surg. 2021;69:228–30. Available from: https://doi.org/
12. Zhang H, Huang S, Xia H, Shi L, Zeng X, Jiang J, et al. The role of peroral endoscopic myotomy for Zenker's diverticulum: a systematic review and meta-analysis. Surg Endosc. 2022;36(5):2749–59. Available from: https://pubmed.ncbi.nlm.nih.gov/35020054/
13. Spadaccini M, Maselli R, Chandrasekar VT, Patel HK, Fugazza A, Galtieri PA, et al. Submucosal tunnelling techniques for Zenker's diverticulum: a systematic review of early outcomes with pooled analysis. Eur J Gastroenterol Hepatol. 2021;33(Suppl 1):E78–83. Available from: https://pubmed.ncbi.nlm.nih.gov/34907984/
14. Al Ghamdi SS, Farha J, Moran RA, Pioche M, Moll F, Yang DJ, et al. Zenker's peroral endoscopic myotomy, or flexible or rigid septotomy for Zenker's diverticulum: a multicenter retrospective comparison. Endoscopy. 2022;54(4):345–51. Available from: https://pubmed.ncbi.nlm.nih.gov/34198355/

Chapter 11
Gastric Peroral Endoscopic Myotomy (G-POEM)/Peroral Pyloromyotomy

Jerry T. Dang and Matthew Kroh

Background

- Gastroparesis is a chronic gastrointestinal condition with increasing prevalence manifested by delayed gastric emptying without mechanical obstruction. Symptoms may include nausea, vomiting, early satiety, abdominal pain, bloating, and weight loss. The prevalence is 267 per 100,000 persons and is twice as common in females [1].
- The mechanism of gastroparesis is a result of gastric motility dysfunction involving impaired antral contractions and incomplete relaxation of the pyloric sphincter. Some proposed contributing factors are neuromuscular dysfunction, hormonal imbalances, and inflammation.
- Etiologies include long-standing diabetes, postsurgical complications related to vagal nerve injury (fundoplication, gastrectomy), idiopathic, medications, connective tissue disorders, neurological disorders, and autoimmune diseases.
- Noninvasive treatments include dietary modifications such as consuming small, frequent meals which are low in fat and fiber accompanied by adequate hydration. Prokinetic medications such as metoclopramide, erythromycin, or domperidone stimulate stomach contractions to promote gastric emptying. These medications may be accompanied by antiemetics.
- Invasive treatments include implantable gastric stimulation devices, which initiate stomach contractions with electrical impulse. Botulinum toxin injection temporarily paralyzes the pyloric sphincter muscles though it has limited effectiveness and short duration and it is poorly supported by data. Pyloric balloon dilation has

J. T. Dang · M. Kroh (✉)
Department of General Surgery, Digestive Disease Institute, Cleveland Clinic, Cleveland, OH, USA
e-mail: DANGJ3@ccf.org; KROHM@ccf.org

M. Ujiki, Z. M. Callahan (eds.), *Third Space Endoscopy*, https://doi.org/10.1007/978-3-031-84509-3_11

also been described. Surgical treatment includes laparoscopic pyloromyotomy, pyloroplasty, and subtotal gastrectomy.

- Conventional treatments of gastroparesis have limitations. Prokinetic medications often have limited efficacy and potential side effects. Gastric electrical stimulation may not provide adequate symptom relief for all patients and device implantation is required. Invasive surgical options (e.g., pyloroplasty, gastrectomy) carry higher risk and morbidity [2].
- Gastric peroral endoscopic myotomy (G-POEM) is a minimally invasive, endoscopic procedure targeting the pyloric sphincter to improve gastric emptying. It is adapted from the POEM (peroral endoscopic myotomy) technique, initially developed for achalasia treatment. G-POEM was first performed by Dr. Mouen A. Khashab in 2013 at Johns Hopkins University [3].
- G-POEM has reduced risk and lower morbidity compared to surgery while preserving gastric anatomy and function. The procedure is usually done as an outpatient and recovery is minimal. It is cost-effective compared to other treatments, such as repeat endoscopic botulinum toxin injections or surgical interventions.
- There is growing evidence in support of G-POEM with an increasing number of studies and case series demonstrating the safety and efficacy of G-POEM for gastroparesis [4]. Concomitant with emerging evidence, there is increasing adoption by expert endoscopists and specialized centers for the management of refractory gastroparesis [5].

Indications

- G-POEM may be indicated in patients with persistent symptoms despite conservative management. These patients may have inadequate response to dietary modifications and prokinetics with significant impact on quality of life or even malnutrition and dehydration.

Patient Evaluation

Initial Evaluation

- Patients are evaluated with a comprehensive medical history and physical examination. Particular attention is paid to reviewing prior diagnostic tests and treatment attempts. It is important to assess comorbidities and overall health status as well as identify potential contraindications to endoscopic procedures. A careful assessment of gastrointestinal anatomy including surgical history should be completed.

- Optimization of medical conditions is paramount such as glycemic control in diabetic patients, management of other gastrointestinal disorders (e.g., reflux, irritable bowel syndrome), adjustment of medications that may affect gastric emptying or increase bleeding risk, and nutritional supplementation if required.

Diagnostic Studies

- The gold standard diagnostic test is gastric emptying scintigraphy which measures stomach contents at the time of ingestion then at 2 and 4 h. Delayed emptying is defined as retention of greater than 60% at 2 hours or greater than 10% at 4 h. Extending the test to 4 h is highly recommended as it increases test sensitivity.
- Other testing includes a wireless motility capsule, antroduodenal manometry, and 13 °C breath tests, though these are less frequently used.
- Careful endoscopy must be performed to exclude mechanical obstruction. This may be accompanied by contrast studies.

Preoperative Preparation

- Collaboration between gastroenterologists, surgeons, dietitians, and other healthcare professionals ensures appropriate patient selection and comprehensive preoperative evaluation.
- Anticoagulant and antiplatelet medications should be discontinued per institutional guidelines, and antibiotic prophylaxis may be given.
- Patients are placed on a clear liquid diet for 1 or more days, depending on severity of gastroparesis and should be fasting for a minimum of 6 h before the procedure.

Technique [6]

Planning

- G-POEM requires a high-definition gastroscope with a large working channel. Endoscopic accessories may include an electrosurgical knife (e.g., Triangle Tip Knife, IT Knife), submucosal injection needle (e.g., DualKnife), hemostatic forceps (e.g., Coagrasper), or endoscopic clips (e.g., QuickClip, Resolution Clip).
- The endoscopic dissection cap may be secured to gastroscope tip with electrical tape (Fig. 11.1).

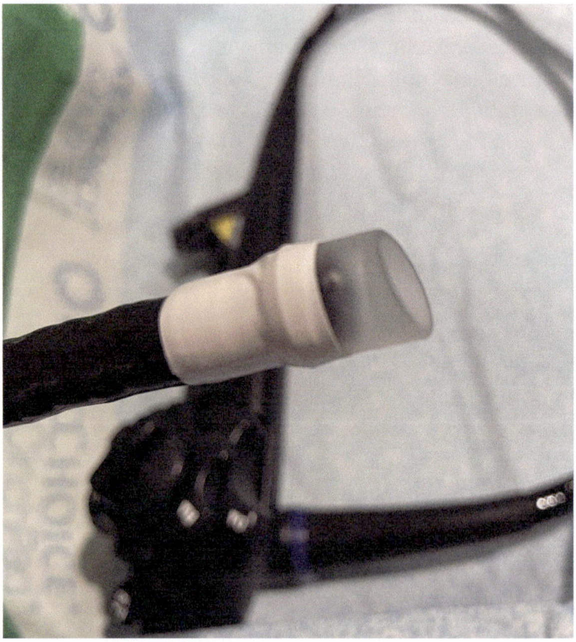

Fig. 11.1 Transparent endoscopic dissection cap secured with electrical tape

- Carbon dioxide insufflation is used to minimize post-procedure abdominal discomfort and reduce the risk of gas-related complications.
- Electrosurgical generator is required with various cutting and coagulation settings (e.g., ERBE VIO, Olympus ESG-400).

Endoscopic Access and Anatomical Landmarks

- The patient is placed supine under general anesthesia with endotracheal intubation.
- The endoscope advanced through the mouth and esophagus, into the stomach, under direct visualization and a thorough inspection of the stomach and pylorus is performed to identify any abnormalities or anatomical variations, such as prepyloric gastric folds, which may impact the procedure.

Submucosal Injection and Mucosal Lifting

- A mucosal entry point is created in the lesser curve, approximately 2–3 cm proximal to the pylorus.

- An injection of a solution (e.g., saline with methylene blue) is used to lift the mucosa and create a submucosal bleb, which provides a cushion and facilitates safe dissection (Fig. 11.2). Alternatively, a submucosal injection needle with a water jet function (e.g., HybridKnife) can be used to create the bleb without the need for separate injection.

Mucosal Incision and Tunnel Creation

- A mucosotomy is made using an electrosurgical knife at the mucosal entry point, with the cutting mode set at an appropriate power output for precise and controlled dissection (Fig. 11.3).
- A submucosal tunnel is created toward the pylorus, using the electrosurgical knife in conjunction with a transparent cap fitted on the endoscope tip for improved visualization and dissection (Fig. 11.4). This can be done using cutting or coagulation modes.
- The tunnel is extended through the pyloric ring into the duodenal bulb, taking care to maintain a safe distance from the underlying muscular layer to avoid perforation (Fig. 11.5).

Pyloric Myotomy

- The pyloric sphincter muscles are identified within the submucosal tunnel, and careful attention is given to distinguish between circular and longitudinal fibers.

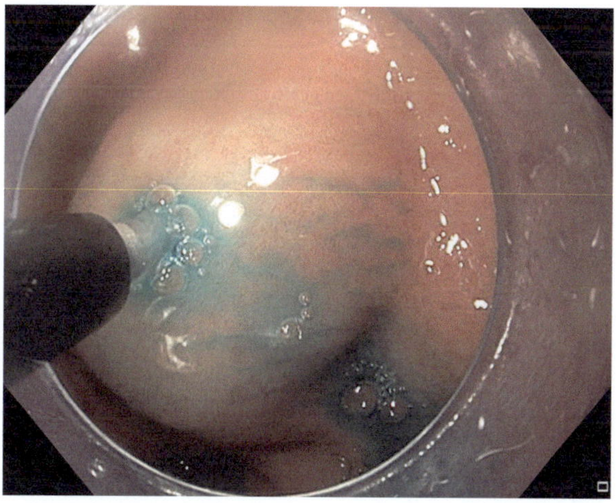

Fig. 11.2 Injection of methylene blue to create to lift mucosa and create submucosal bleb

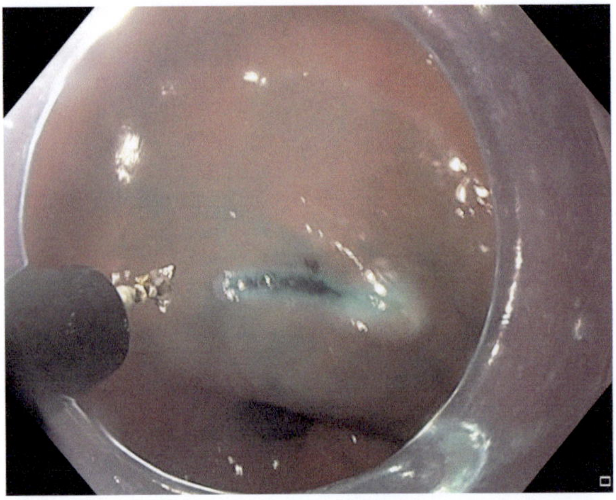

Fig. 11.3 Mucosotomy using triangle tip electrosurgical knife

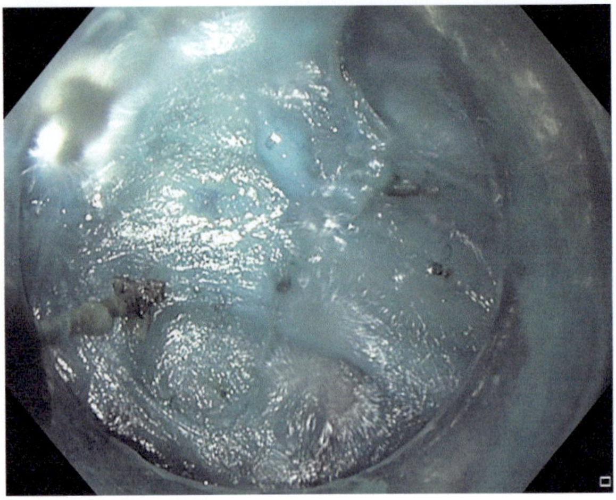

Fig. 11.4 Submucosal tunneling using electrosurgical knife and transparent cap

- A selective myotomy of the circular muscle fibers is performed using the electrosurgical knife, with the cutting or coagulation mode set at an appropriate power output to ensure adequate hemostasis during the procedure (Fig. 11.6).
- The myotomy is extended from the gastric antrum, through the pyloric ring, and into the proximal duodenum, ensuring that the cut extends at least into the duodenum to achieve optimal results.
- Intentional preservation of the longitudinal muscle fibers is performed to prevent perforation and maintain the integrity of the gastric and duodenal walls.

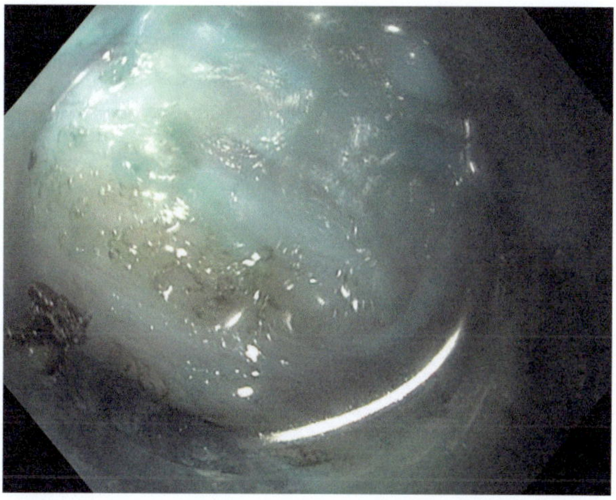

Fig. 11.5 Tunnel created under the pylorus

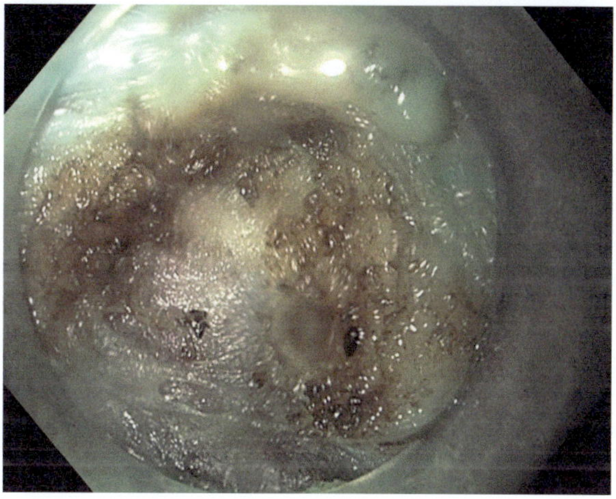

Fig. 11.6 Completed pyloromyotomy

Closure of the Mucosal Entry Point

- The submucosal tunnel is inspected for adequate hemostasis, with the use of cautery or hemostatic forceps if active bleeding is encountered.
- The mucosal incision is closed using endoscopic clips, ensuring complete closure to prevent leakage of gastric contents and potential complications such as peritonitis or abscess formation (Fig. 11.7).
- Application of additional clips or sutures may be used, if necessary, to achieve a secure closure.

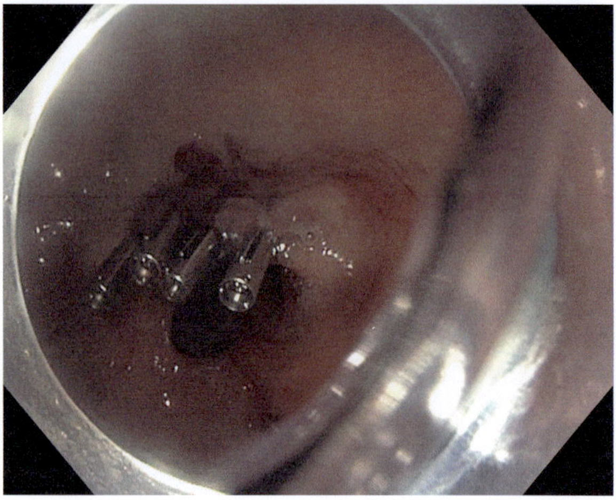

Fig. 11.7 Closure of mucosotomy with endoscopic clips

Technique Variations

- The mucosotomy and submucosal tunneling may be done along the greater curvature. This can be more difficult but may be necessary for repeat G-POEM for patients who have had previous lesser curve G-POEM.
- Endoscopic suturing devices (e.g., OverStitch) for closure of the mucosal entry point may be performed. However, endoscopic suturing devices are more expensive with similar complication rates [7].
- Intraoperative endoscopic ultrasound (EUS) may be used to assess the depth of myotomy and ensure adequate division of the circular muscle fibers.

Training and Proficiency

- G-POEM requires advanced endoscopic skills, including submucosal dissection and endoscopic suturing or clipping.
- Gastroenterologists or surgeons performing G-POEM should have prior experience with endoscopic submucosal dissection (ESD) and peroral endoscopic myotomy (POEM) procedures.
- Training in specialized centers and participation in dedicated courses or workshops is recommended to ensure proficiency and minimize the risk of complications.

Postoperative Care

- Immediate postoperative monitoring includes close observation for early signs of complications, such as bleeding, perforation, or infection.
- Patients are typically discharged on the same day if tolerating clear fluids.
- The postoperative diet includes clear liquids within a few hours after the procedure, as tolerated. Patients are then kept on full liquids for 1–2 weeks and then progress to a soft diet and then a regular diet over the next few days, depending on patient tolerance and physician recommendations.
- Postoperative medications include proton pump inhibitors (PPIs) or histamine-2 receptor antagonists (H2RAs) to reduce gastric acid production and promote mucosal healing as well as sucralfate twice a day for a month to encourage mucosal healing.
- Anticoagulant and antiplatelet medications are resumed per institutional guidelines and individual patient risk factors.
- Consultation with a dietitian is helpful to develop a personalized nutrition plan and assist in continuation of the preoperative gastroparesis diet.

Outcomes [8–10]

- Most patients experience a significant reduction in symptoms, such as nausea, vomiting, early satiety, and abdominal pain, as well as improved quality of life with decreased reliance on medications. However, there is a potential for recurrence of symptoms or need for additional interventions in a subset of patients.
- There are high technical and clinical success rates reported in various studies, with success rates ranging from 70% to 90% for symptom improvement and gastric emptying. These rates are comparable or superior to outcomes of other treatment options, such as endoscopic pyloric injection of botulinum toxin or surgical intervention (e.g., pyloroplasty).
- G-POEM may be more cost-effective than alternative treatments, such as repeat endoscopic botulinum toxin injections or surgical interventions, due to reduced need for additional interventions and hospitalizations [11].
- There is a low overall complication rate associated with G-POEM [12]; complications include bleeding, perforation, ulceration, and capnoperitoneum. The risk of perforation is generally low and can be effectively managed with a combination of antibiotics and, if required, endoscopic or surgical intervention. Ulcers may form at the site of incision and myotomy but usually heal spontaneously with proton pump inhibitor therapy. Capnoperitoneum is often self-resolving and rarely necessitates intervention. In cases causing respiratory symptoms, a simple decompression with a 14-gauge needle can alleviate symptoms.
- G-POEM has a lower complication rate and shorter length of stay than laparoscopic pyloroplasty [13].

Pearls	Pitfalls
Patient selection	Select appropriate patients for G-POEM based on comprehensive evaluation and indications. Inadequate patient selection may lead to suboptimal outcomes or increased risk of complications
Proficiency	Ensure proficiency in advanced endoscopic techniques, including submucosal dissection. Inadequate training or experience may result in increased risk of complications during the procedure
Insufflation	Use carbon dioxide insufflation to minimize post-procedure abdominal discomfort. Air insufflation may cause increased discomfort and risk of gas-related complications
Mucosal lift	Create a clear submucosal bleb to facilitate safe dissection and tunnel creation. Insufficient mucosal lifting may lead to increased risk of perforation during tunnel creation
Longitudinal fibers	Preserve the longitudinal muscle fibers during pyloric myotomy. Injury to longitudinal muscle fibers may result in perforation or compromised gastric and duodenal integrity
Closure	Achieve complete closure of the mucosal entry point to prevent leakage and complications. Incomplete closure may lead to leakage, peritonitis, or abscess formation
Postoperative monitoring	Monitor patients closely for early signs of complications postoperatively. Delayed detection of complications may result in worsened patient outcomes

References

1. Ye Y, Yin Y, Huh SY, Almansa C, Bennett D, Camilleri M. Epidemiology, etiology, and treatment of gastroparesis: real-world evidence from a large US national claims database. Gastroenterology. 2022;162(1):109–21.
2. Camilleri M, Kuo B, Nguyen L, Vaughn VM, Petrey J, Greer K, et al. ACG clinical guideline: gastroparesis. Am J Gastroenterol. 2022;117(8):1197–220.
3. Khashab MA, Stein E, Clarke JO, Saxena P, Kumbhari V, Chander Roland B, et al. Gastric peroral endoscopic myotomy for refractory gastroparesis: first human endoscopic pyloromyotomy (with video). Gastrointest Endosc. 2013;78(5):764–8.
4. Aghaie Meybodi M, Qumseya B, Shakoor D, Lobner K, Vosoughi K, Ichkhanian Y, et al. Efficacy and feasibility of G-POEM in management of patients with refractory gastroparesis: a systematic review and meta-analysis. Endosc Int Open. 2019;07(03):E322–9.
5. Haisley KR, Swanström LL. The modern age of POEM: the past, present and future of per-oral endoscopic myotomy. J Gastrointest Surg. 2021;25(2):551–7.
6. Allemang MT, Strong AT, Haskins IN, Rodriguez J, Ponsky JL, Kroh M. How I do it: per-Oral Pyloromyotomy (POP). J Gastrointest Surg. 2017;21(11):1963–8.
7. Hustak R, Vackova Z, Krajciova J, Kieslichova JSE, Jan JM. Endoscopic clips versus overstitch suturing system device for mucosotomy closure after peroral endoscopic pyloromyotomy (G - POEM): a prospective single - center study. Surg Endosc. 2022;36(12):9254–61.
8. Rodriguez J, Strong AT, Haskins IN, Landreneau JP, Allemang MT, El-Hayek K, et al. Per-oral Pyloromyotomy (POP) for medically refractory gastroparesis: short term results from the first 100 patients at a high volume center. Ann Surg. 2018;268(3):421–30.
9. Vosoughi K, Ichkhanian Y, Benias P, Miller L, Aadam AA, Triggs JR, et al. Gastric per- oral endoscopic myotomy (G-POEM) for refractory gastroparesis: results from an international prospective trial. Gut. 2022;71(1):25–33.

10. Abdelfatah MM, Noll A, Kapil N, Shah R, Li L, Nustas R, et al. Long-term outcome of gastric per-Oral endoscopic Pyloromyotomy in treatment of gastroparesis. Clin Gastroenterol Hepatol. 2021;19(4):816–24.
11. Abdelfatah MM, Noll A, Kapil N, Shah R, Li L, Nustas R, et al. Long-term outcome of gastric per-Oral endoscopic Pyloromyotomy in treatment of gastroparesis. Clin Gastroenterol Hepatol. 2021;19(4):816–24. Available from: https://pubmed.ncbi.nlm.nih.gov/32450364/
12. Tan J, Shrestha SM, Wei M, Wang P, Shi J, Lu Y, et al. Feasibility, safety, and long-term efficacy of gastric peroral endoscopic myotomy (G-POEM) for postsurgical gastroparesis: a single-center and retrospective study of a prospective database. Surg Endosc. 2021;35(7):3459–70. Available from: https://link.springer.com/article/10.1007/s00464-020-07793-0
13. Landreneau JP, Strong AT, El-Hayek K, Tu C, Villamere J, Ponsky JL, et al. Laparoscopic pyloroplasty versus endoscopic per-oral pyloromyotomy for the treatment of gastroparesis. Surg Endosc. 2019;33(3):773–81. Available from: https://pubmed.ncbi.nlm.nih.gov/30019220/

Index

M. Ujiki, Z. M. Callahan (eds.), *Third Space Endoscopy*,
https://doi.org/10.1007/978-3-031-84509-3